A Beginner's Guide to Critical Thinking and Writing in Health and Social Care

Helen Aveyard, Pam Sharp and Mary Woolliams

Open University Press

Open University Press
McGraw-Hill Education
McGraw-Hill House
Shoppenhangers Road
Maidenhead
Berkshire
England
SL6 2QL

email: enquiries@openup.co.uk
world wide web: www.openup.co.uk

and Two Penn Plaza, New York, NY 10121-2289, USA

First published 2011

A catalogue record of this book is available from the British Library

ISBN-13: 978-0-33-524366-2 (pb)
ISBN-10: 0-33-524366-5 (pb)
eISBN: 978-0-33-524367-9

Library of Congress Cataloging-in-Publication Data
CIP data applied for

Typeset by RefineCatch Limited, Bungay, Suffolk
Printed and bound by CPI Group (UK) Ltd, Croydon, CR0 4YY

Fictitious names of companies, products, people, characters and/or data that may be used herein (in case studies or in examples) are not intended to represent any real individual, company, product or event.

The *McGraw·Hill* Companies

Contents

In this chapter we will:

- Introduce and define critical thinking and say why it is important.
- Give an example of critical thinking in action.
- Introduce 'six questions to trigger critical thinking'.
- Explore why critical thinking has become more important in recent years.
- Explore how critical thinking can help you in your academic assignments and professional decision-making.

In this chapter we will:

- Identify what is readily available information.
- Discuss how to judge the quality and usefulness of this information.
- Show how you can begin to think critically about the information you find and how to use it.

In this chapter we will:

- Explain why you need to dig a little deeper to find the 'best available' evidence.

- Explore why critical thinking is important for developing a broader perspective in your personal, professional and academic life.
- Discuss the changes influencing health and social care in the twenty-first century, and explore ways to respond to these as a critical thinker.
- Describe what qualities and skills are needed to think critically from a broader perspective in relation to health and social care.
- Discuss how you can broaden your horizons through networking with professionals and academics in different disciplines, professions and specialist fields.

About the authors

Helen Aveyard (BSc, RGN, MA, PGDip, PhD) is a senior lecturer at Oxford Brookes University and author of the best selling-book *Doing a Literature Review in Health and Social Care* (second edition, 2010) and *A Beginner's Guide to Evidence Based Practice* (2009), both published by Open University Press. Helen has also published widely on informed consent and nursing care procedures and has authored book chapters in health care ethics and research. Prior to her lectureship post, Helen undertook doctoral study at the University of London. http://shsc.brookes.ac.uk/dr-helen-aveyard

Pam Sharp (MSc, PGDip RGN) is a senior lecturer at Oxford Brookes University. She is co-author of *A Beginner's Guide to Evidence Based Practice* (2009), published by Open University Press. She runs an undergraduate evidence-based practice module and teaches critical appraisal of research in Hong Kong. She has previously contributed chapters to the third and fourth editions of Bulman and Schutz, *Reflective Practice in Nursing* (Blackwell, 2004, 2008). She has particular interests in practice education and mentoring. http://shsc.brookes.ac.uk/pam-sharp

Mary Woolliams qualified as a nurse and health visitor in 1990, then specialized in acute general medical nursing and the care of older people. In 2003 Mary joined the School of Health and Social Care at Oxford Brookes University as a senior lecturer in adult nursing, and more recently she has taken on leadership of one of the interprofessional learning modules for the pre-qualifying programmes. Mary has also been involved in a variety of projects within the university aiming to assist students to develop their study skills, including developing some popular practical resources and guides. http://shsc.brookes.ac.uk/mary-woolliams

Introduction

This book is for you if you are:

- A student undertaking a pre-registration course in any of the health and social care professions.
- A registered practitioner, who may be returning to post-qualifying study after a career break.

It is also for:

- Anyone who feels that they are not sure what to believe when they read conflicting professional information.
- Those who tend to take things at 'face value', and need to dig deeper into the evidence they come across.
- Practice assessors or mentors[1] who are supporting students/learners in practice and are aware of the need to be more critical of the information and evidence they use.

You may already know that:

- There is a large amount and many types of information available, and this is of variable quality.
- You need to be able to make sense of the information that you use in practice and in your academic writing.
- Some findings from one source may conflict with those of another.

---

[1] The term practice assessor/mentor will be used throughout to describe those who support learners in practice. A variety of other terms are used throughout the professions to mean the same thing, such as clinical educator, supervisor, practice educator/teacher, clinical tutor or instructor.

- You are legally and professionally accountable for your practice once you are a registered practitioner and need to use information appropriately.
- You cannot defend your practice by saying 'I was told to do it this way'.

So . . . where do you start?
You might feel that you do not know where to begin when it comes to being critical of what you read, see or hear. Life would be easy if we could believe everything without the need to judge its quality. Furthermore, there is simply so much information available. Making sense of the information and evidence you encounter can seem daunting.

This book will help you to understand and be more critical of the information you read, see or hear in a jargon-free way.

Aim of the book

The aim of this book is to help you develop skills in critical thinking; that is, not accepting everything you read, see and hear at face value but instead making sense of the information you use in your professional and/or university work. There is such a vast amount of information out there that, without these skills, it is difficult to know what to include in your academic assignments or how to incorporate new information into your practice. It is easy to feel overwhelmed and you may find that you make decisions in your professional practice or write academic assignments based on inappropriate evidence; bad choices about professional practice are likely to be made which can have a deep impact on patients and clients. This in turn can have a significant impact on both your practice and academic work. Critical thinking in writing and practice is a vital skill that all students/learners and professionals need to acquire from the very start of their practice experience and in their writing.

Furthermore, your ability to be critical will be assessed and this is a substantial component in almost all marking criteria for those studying for a professional qualification in health and social care. In fact, 'being critical' is probably the key element of all higher education courses.

How to get the most from this book

- We recommend that you begin at the beginning and work through the book systematically, as the material is presented in the order in which we think it should be read.

- You can use the index if you have a particular issue you want to find out about.
- Use the glossary for explanations of words you are unfamiliar with.
- Work with a colleague or a student/learner who is more confident in critical thinking in practice.
- Get access to the internet and start 'searching' using relevant databases (don't leave it until you really need to find information quickly).
- Be more critical of sources of information you come across on a daily basis.
- Don't give up if you find something difficult or don't understand it. Feel good about every new thing that you have learned.

Structure of the book

In the first chapter we discuss the concept of critical thinking and why it is important. In Chapter 2 we will consider the best response to 'readily available information'; by this we mean information that you encounter on an everyday basis and do not need to look too hard to find. In Chapter 3 we explore how you should 'dig a bit deeper' for evidence when you need to, using comprehensive searching strategies. In Chapters 4 and 5 we discuss in more detail how to use critical thinking skills in your written academic work, presentations and in practice, and in Chapter 6 we consider the broader implications of critical thinking within health and social care.

We will use these terms

Critical analysis: this is when you break down or explore in depth all the information available relating to an issue or question. This may involve exploring what is happening and the reasons why. You may need to consider and access alternative perspectives including theory.

Critical appraisal: this is when you consider the strengths and limitations of each piece of evidence you use.

Critical thinking: this is when you adopt a questioning approach and thoughtful attitude to what you read, see or hear, rather than accept things at face value. It relates to both academic work and professional practice.

Health or social care professional: this includes: nurses, midwives, doctors, occupational therapists, physiotherapists, operating department practitioners, dieticians, paramedics, radiographers, speech and language therapists, art therapists, chiropodists/podiatrists, clinical scientists, orthoptists, prosthetists, social care workers, orthotists, osteopaths.

Patient/client: this is used to refer to all service users that health and social care professionals may come into contact with. Although not stated you may also need to consider carers' perspectives.

Practice assessor/mentor: this is used to describe those who support learners in practice.

Students/learners: this is used to refer to anyone, pre- or post-qualifying, who may be undertaking study either formally or informally.

Examples

We have tried to include examples that may be easily understood by a range of professions, as we all work within a wider team. We can learn a lot from the richness and diversity of examples from other professional groups even if they do not directly apply to our practice.

Web addresses

We have in places given you web addresses which were correct and accessible at the time of publication but do sometimes change. You may need to input the organization's details and search within their site if the address no longer works.

Use the symbols

 Key information

 Activity for you to do

 Think point

1

What is 'critical thinking' and why is it important?

Introduction to critical thinking: what it is and why it is important in health and social care • Defining critical thinking • Is critical thinking a new idea? • Critical thinking is not as common as you may think • An example of critical thinking in action • How you can think more critically – using 'six questions to trigger critical thinking' • The need to think critically has never been more important . . . • How critical thinking can help you in your academic assignments and professional decision-making • In summary • Key points

In this chapter we will:

- Introduce and define critical thinking and say why it is important.
- Give an example of critical thinking in action.
- Introduce 'six questions to trigger critical thinking'.
- Explore why critical thinking has become more important in recent years.
- Explore how critical thinking can help you in your academic assignments and professional decision-making.

Introduction to critical thinking: what it is and why it is important in health and social care

In short, critical thinking is about taking a step back and thinking logically and carefully about the information you have, rather than believing everything you read, see and hear. Critical thinking is about questioning and evaluating the information available to you.

Critical thinking is probably what you already do when you read a newspaper. You question what you read and often take what you read with a 'pinch of salt'. There is often good reason for this. Take the headline 'Freddie Starr Ate My Hamster' from *The Sun* newspaper back in 1986 which created much publicity, but the facts behind the headline were hotly disputed (Starr 2001). Critical thinking is probably also something you already do when you listen to and take part in discussions in your day-to-day life. You listen and probably join in, but inside you start wondering if there is any evidence behind the claims being made or whether it is all 'hype'. Or maybe you are not always critical of what you read, see and hear. Sometimes our own experiences make us biased and prevent us from being logical. To give an extreme **example**: someone who has just survived a plane crash is likely to perceive plane travel as dangerous, even though it is often quoted to be the safest form of travel. There are many times when we need to examine our perceptions and biases if we want to make logical choices. You may have heard of the term **reflection**. We discuss this in more detail in Chapters 4 and 5 but in principle when you take the time to reflect you consider your thoughts and feelings and how they impact on the decisions you make.

 Consider what preconceived ideas and misconceptions about everyday life might affect what you think, do, and how you do it.

You might think that in professional life, everybody is rational; that professional literature and conversations you hear among professionals are different and you can believe all that you read, see and hear. Unfortunately this is not always the case. Even professional literature varies a lot in quality and it is essential that you can make sense of what you read. There is also a vast amount of evidence, some of it good and some less good. The quality of the dialogue you hear in professional practice will also vary.

The implications of this within health and social care are enormous. Kamhi (2011) describes how false beliefs that we develop can lead to the making of wrong or badly judged decisions. In other words, if we are not critical of the beliefs we hold, this can lead to poor decision-making. In our personal lives, we take the consequences of this ourselves. In our professional life, it is our patients and clients who will be affected if our care is based on false beliefs.

Imagine you experienced severe sickness many years ago when you were given the pain-killing drug morphine after an operation. You were intolerant of the drug and this is an extreme side effect that affects a very small proportion of people who receive the drug. Now, as a practitioner, you do not routinely offer the drug even though it is written up 'as required' and you try to dissuade people from consenting to this drug, even when they are in severe pain and morphine is the drug of choice. In this situation, lack of critical thinking can lead to the delivery of inappropriate care. This is an example of how a false belief can lead to a badly judged decision.

or

Imagine you are a social worker who experienced severe bullying as a child at nursery school. You now find yourself reluctant to advise mothers in your care to send their children to nursery even when the social situation recommends that this is the best arrangement for the child concerned.

Kida (2006) provides a summary of the most common thinking errors. These include: being persuaded by *personal experience* rather than objective evidence and preferring *evidence that supports our ideas* rather than objective evidence. Critical thinking, and in particular using reflection (as we discuss in Chapters 4 and 5), helps us to avoid these thinking errors. Critical thinking involves taking a step back and thinking logically about the evidence that you have. Facione (1990: 2) explains why critical thinking is important:

> *Critical thinking is essential as a tool of inquiry. As such, critical thinking is a liberating force in education and a powerful resource in one's personal and civic life. While not synonymous with good thinking, critical thinking is a pervasive and self-rectifying human phenomenon.*

This is very important in health and social care. You cannot help bringing your own experiences with you into practice. What is important is that you acknowledge these and examine your beliefs in a critical way. You will hear a large amount of professional dialogue and have access to a vast amount of professional literature, and you need to work out what is useful and relevant and what is not; you need to make sure you are using reliable information wisely, both in your academic assignments and to inform your practice. In this book we will explain how you do this.

Defining critical thinking

There are many definitions of critical thinking, but if you look at them carefully the message is largely consistent.

Price and Harrington (2010: 8) have recently defined critical thinking as the gathering, sifting, synthesizing and evaluating of information which enables the practitioner to act as a:

> *knowledgeable doer – someone who selects, combines, judges and uses information in order to proceed in a professional manner.*

Wade and Tarvis (2008: 7) define critical thinking as:

> *the ability to assess claims and make objective judgements on the basis of well supported reasons and evidence rather than emotion and anecdote. Critical thinkers are able to look for flaws in argument and resist claims that have no support.*

In other words, if you are a critical thinker, you think carefully about what you read, see and hear. When you hear a news story or listen to a discussion among friends, you question the quality of the evidence and the conclusions drawn from that evidence. If the topic is important to you, you endeavour to find out more information which will help to make sense of the facts. This enables you to form an overall view and then apply it to the situation at hand.

Have you been a critical thinker in the past?

Refer back to how you have used information in the past and consider the potential problems with your approach. Did you:

- Scan read written information?
- Only use readily available sources?
- Ignore research that didn't agree with your current practice?
- Listen to advice from colleagues without questioning?
- Copy what you observed without question?
- Believe everything that you read without questioning the authority of the writers or the quality of the arguments or evidence?
- Use only one or two sources?
- Only use sources that supported your view?

Or do you feel that you consider the merits of each piece of information you come across and seek out further resources or opinions when the available information does not seem to be complete? We need to ensure that we take into account all the facts before making judgements. This helps us personally and professionally to ensure we make considered and reflective decisions, considering the relevant evidence and not just following the actions of others.

Is critical thinking a new idea?

Critical thinking is not a new idea in health and social care and many professionals have always questioned what they read, see and hear. The ancient roots of critical thinking date back to the ideas of the Greek philosopher Socrates, who is credited with pioneering a questioning and rational approach to problem-solving and encouraging people to reject statements made on the basis of confused meaning and inadequate evidence. We can see then that the concept of critical thinking has stood the test of time, however, as shown by **Examples 1** and **2** below, the the concept is neither universally nor routinely applied.

Example 1: evidence of a lack of critical thinking

Take **for example** a recent media story which was running in early January 2011. Newspaper and television reports (*Daily Mail, The Guardian, The Daily Telegraph, Channel 4 News*, 3–6 January 2011) documented that:

hundreds of women have become pregnant whilst using a particular contraceptive device

Almost every newspaper and news programme in the UK carried this story at this time. The reports carried the news that 584 women had become pregnant while using the 'Implanon' contraceptive device. While these numbers are not disputed and many women may well have got pregnant while using the device, what the report didn't tell us was the overall context – that is how many women used the device in total and hence whether the failure rate was higher than would be expected (given that no contraception is 100 per cent effective). Media reports implied that the number of unwanted pregnancies associated with this device was excessively high and exceeded the number of unwanted pregnancies associated with other contraceptive devices. Yet when Radio 4's *More or Less* picked up this story on 7 January 2011, it was set in context. Despite the stated number of pregnancies associated with the device, researchers for the programme quoted a failure rate for Implanon of 0.06 per cent – far lower than any other commonly used method including sterilization, providing evidence that the device remains one of the most effective ways of preventing pregnancy. This would seem to be a clear example of statistics being represented in a misleading way, and illustrates perfectly why it is so important to be critical of what you read and to look beyond the headlines of a newspaper report.

Critical thinking requires that you look beyond the initial headline that catches your eye. In the examples cited above, critical thinking was required to question the source of the evidence and look further afield, considering the huge numbers of people *successfully* using the device compared to those experiencing problems.

Example 2: further evidence of a lack of critical thinking

The controversy over the measles, mumps and rubella vaccination (MMR) gives us another good example of why it is so important to be critical of what you read, see and hear – in other words, to critically appraise. The original research by Wakefield *et al.* (1998) was hugely influential.

This research paper has now been retracted by the publishing journal, *The Lancet*. This was because the evidence presented was later found to be flawed. However, before it was retracted, it attracted wide publicity. The paper described how 12 children who had received the MMR vaccination also went on to develop either autism or bowel disease. Yet millions of children have had the MMR vaccination and suffered no ill effects. Also, children who have *not* been given the MMR vaccination have developed autism and/or bowel disease. Anyone looking critically at Wakefield *et al.*'s paper can see that the evidence it provides is not strong; in fact it is very weak indeed, and as in the previous example, critical thinking is required to consider the method in which the data about the vaccination was collected and presented. A critical thinker would have used rational judgement and critical appraisal to explore the quality of the paper and to expose its weaknesses. Yet somehow, this paper was so well publicized, and not critically evaluated, that vaccination rates plummeted as parents feared for the safety of the vaccination. In a further twist to this story, not only was the study very weak, but much later on it was found to be fraudulent – there is evidence that the details of some of the 12 children described in the study were fabricated (Deer 2011).

Critical thinking is not as common as you may think

Having read Examples 1 and 2, you might not be surprised to read that we argue that critical thinking is not as common as we might like to think (which is why we have written this book). We have given the examples of the misleading newspaper headlines and misinterpreted poor quality journal article. Indeed there is evidence that many professionals do not always think critically about the evidence they use. When researchers (Petrovic *et al.* 2001) undertook a survey of health care providers to establish whether their practice had changed in the light of the MMR vaccination scare, they found that a large number of health care professionals expressed reservations about giving the vaccination because of Wakefield *et al.*'s study. This suggests that these health care professionals had either not read or thought critically about the evidence relating to this aspect of their practice.

Unfortunately there are many other such examples. On his 'Bad Science' website (www.badscience.net) and in his book, Goldacre (2009) illustrates what can happen when people are not critical of information that is presented to them; he explores many commonly held ideas about popular culture, most of which involve health and social care. Using a critical approach, he examines the minimal evidence on which many of these ideas are based and yet which attract huge popular interest. **For example:** so called 'miracle cures' such as herbal remedies or fruit drinks are advertised and sold and yet the evidence underpinning their medicinal qualities is often unproven. Goldacre is particularly vocal on the 'science' of detoxification and outlines the lack of good quality evidence proving any benefits of this widely used practice. Goldacre's examples illustrate how 'weighing up' or critical appraisal of the evidence has not been carried out and as a result many people are adhering to practices or beliefs that have no scientific underpinning. In other words, there is very little evidence behind some of these popular 'remedies' and it is important that people think critically and question this, rather than take at face value the claims made by those who will profit financially from their use.

An example of critical thinking in action

In order to be a critical thinker you need to be able to understand and make sense of what you read, see and hear. As a professional, inundated with a vast amount of information, you are very likely to come across sources of information that conflict with each other. You need to understand why this is the case in order to make sense of what you read, see and hear. This is a long-term goal and you are not expected to understand all the complex information, literature and evidence you come across right from the start. However, if you start off by developing the right skills, you will become more and more able to do this.

In **Example 3**, we consider Facione's (1990: 2) criteria for a critical thinker and apply these to the situation described. Facione describes the characteristics of a critical thinker as being someone who does not accept things at face value:

> *The ideal critical thinker is habitually inquisitive, well-informed, trustful of reason, open-minded, flexible, fair-minded in evaluation, honest in facing personal biases, prudent in making judgements, willing to reconsider, clear about issues, orderly in complex matters, diligent in seeking relevant information, reasonable in the selection of criteria, focused in inquiry, and persistent in seeking results which are as precise as the subject and the circumstances of inquiry permit.*

In **Example 3** we will highlight the characteristics demonstrated from the above quote in **bold**.

Example 3: critical thinking in action

In this example we demonstrate how you can take a critical approach. We will consider the information provided by a letter printed in a health care journal:

Geleijnse, J.M., Brouwer, I.A. and Feskens, E.J.M. (2006) Risks and benefits of omega 3 fats: health benefits of omega 3 fats are in doubt, *British Medical Journal*, 332: 915

We will consider how you should judge the quality of evidence provided by the letter and how you should act on it.

Let's imagine you meet a patient or client who has read a letter which seems to cast doubt on the health benefits of taking omega 3 fat supplements. The patient/client shows you the letter and asks you about the benefit of taking these supplements.

You read the letter. **Inquisitive and open minded**, you remember attending a lecture about food supplements and have heard about the potential benefits of omega 3 fat supplements. You remember that omega 3 fats are used to prevent or alleviate a variety of illnesses. This letter seems to question their benefits. Feeling somewhat confused yourself, you promise to find out more information. You realize you cannot answer your patient/client from the information presented, and demonstrating Facione's requirement of **persistence**, you decide to seek further information in order to be **well informed**.

The first thing to do is to consider the quality of the evidence you have been presented with. Don't be tempted just to accept the headline that you have been shown as fact. You need further information. Indeed Facione tells us to be **diligent in seeking further information**. Remember that a letter – even one printed in a reputable journal – simply represents someone's opinion. It does not provide sufficient evidence upon which to base any firm conclusions although it could trigger further action on your part.

The evidence that is generally most useful in guiding our professional practice is research evidence. We will discuss what research is and how you recognize it in later chapters of this book; however at this stage you can see how a systematic scientific investigation or project (which is generally what research is) is likely to be stronger evidence than someone's views as printed in a letter.

When you read the letter more closely, you discover that it is referring to the use of omega 3 fats for the prevention of cardiovascular disease and cancer in particular. You then read on and discover out that the writers of the letter are referring to a recently published piece of research:

ORIGINAL RESEARCH: Hopper, L. *et al.* (2006) Risks and benefits of omega 3 fats for mortality, cardiovascular disease, and cancer: systematic review, *British Medical Journal*, 332: 752–60.

Given that the letter itself is not good evidence upon which to base your practice, your next step should be to search for and find the article to which the letter is referring using subject-specific search engines (we will discuss how to do this in Chapter 3). This is demonstrating Facione's characteristic of **persistence**.

When you locate the research you find that it is a *systematic review*. A systematic review is usually very strong evidence indeed. Whereas one piece of research gives you results from one study, a review of results looks at the results of all studies that have been undertaken in a particular area. In a systematic review, all the relevant papers that have been published on a particular topic are collated and reviewed so that all the evidence can be seen together – we will discuss more about this approach in the next chapter.

In this case, the researchers examined research which explored the role of omega 3 fats in the prevention of cardiovascular disease, cancer and overall morbidity. The authors concluded that there is little evidence that omega 3 fats play an effective part in the prevention of these diseases. However, when you look at this piece of research in more detail, you find that the researchers included in their review not only studies of omega 3 fats but also of another acid (linolenic acid, a vegetable oil not to be confused with alpha linolenic acid). In other words, the results of studies using non-omega 3 fats were combined with studies of using omega 3 fats only, and the review did not focus solely on omega 3 fats. The finding that there is little evidence that omega 3 fats are effective in prevention of disease is therefore somewhat misleading, as we do not actually know what the findings would have been if omega 3 fats only had been studied, rather than omega 3 fats and linolenic acid. In order to establish the effectiveness of omega 3 fats in the prevention of disease, researchers would need to review research papers relating only to the effects of taking omega 3 fat supplements.

Your response to the patient/client would probably be to explain that the research (systematic review) referred to in the letter was a review of the effects of other substances in addition to omega 3 fats and that we cannot really tell from this review how effective omega 3 fat supplements alone are in this respect. You could go on to say that the benefits of omega 3 fats are still being explored.

From **Example 3**, you can see why it is so important to be a critical thinker and a critical reader. In working through this example, you have demonstrated that you can **make sense of complex issues** (Facione 1990). This enables you to get behind the headlines to see what the evidence is really telling you. You can see how a letter alone is not sufficient evidence upon which to base practice or recommendations to patients or clients. It is important to dig beneath titles and headlines to find out what the information is really about.

How you can think more critically – using 'six questions to trigger critical thinking'

We cannot stress enough how important it is to challenge your own assumptions and consider whether you hold any biases that might affect your views or perspectives on a topic. It is also important to **read** and **ask questions** about what people tell you, and also to **make sense** of what you read, see or hear. You will often come across the following terms:

Critical thinking is when you adopt a questioning approach and thoughtful attitude to what you read, see or hear, rather than accepting things at face value. It relates to both academic work and professional practice. Critical thinking involves a **critical appraisal** *of the information available to you.*

Critical appraisal is when you consider the strengths and limitations of the evidence you read see and hear, depending on the type of evidence you have. The types of questions you need to ask yourself are:

- ***Where** does this information come from?*
- ***What** is being said?*
- ***How** did they write this?*
- ***Who** is telling me this?*
- ***When** was this written?*
- ***Why** has this been written?*

*This means making a judgement about the facts and the quality of evidence on which these facts are based. Critical appraisal involves **critical analysis**.*

*****Critical analysis** is when you break down or explore in depth all the information available relating to an issue or question. This may involve exploring what is happening and the reasons why (see **Examples 1, 2** and **3**). You may need to consider and access alternative perspectives, including theory.*

Introducing our 'six questions to trigger critical thinking'

The following six questions have been adapted from a tool devised by Woolliams *et al.* (2009). You can use these questions to help you consider the

Six questions to trigger critical thinking	
Where did you find the information? Did you just 'come across' it? Or did you access it through a systematic search?	**What** is it and **what** are the key messages or results/findings? Is it a research study, professional opinion, discussion, website or other?
How has the author/speaker come to their conclusions? Is their line of reasoning logical and understandable? If it is research or a review of research, how was it carried out, was it done well and do the conclusions reflect the findings?	**Who** has written/said this? Is the author/speaker an organization or an individual? Are they an expert in the topic? Could they have any bias? How do you know?
When was this written/said? Older key information may still be valid, but you need to check if there has been more recent work.	**Why** has this been written/said? Who is the information aimed at – professionals or patient/client groups? What is the aim of the information?

strengths and weaknesses of any piece of evidence you come across (**for example**: news items, research reports, discussion with colleagues and so on).

You can use these questions as a prompt to help you ask questions about *any* information you have; to make a judgement about its quality and therefore how you use it in your practice or academic work. Unfortunately, there is no exact way to judge the relevance of information – this remains your judgement. However, as a general rule, research studies will provide you with stronger evidence than more anecdotal literature and information from experts will be stronger than information from people with less experience or who are less well known. Also, recent high-quality literature will be stronger than older literature, but no literature is perfect.

Identifying the type of information you use

We suggest that you get used to citing some detail about the information that you use in your academic work and be prepared to present the information in your practice environment. **For example**: if the information you use in an assignment is a research report, say this. If it is anecdotal information or professional opinion, say this as well. This lets your audience know that you are aware of the quality of the literature you use. In general, you can use as many different sources of information as you like in your written work as long as you let the reader know that you are aware of the strengths and weaknesses of each source of information and remember not to use weaker sources to make critical points.

The need to think critically has never been more important . . .

There are two reasons for this. First, there has been a vast increase in our **professional knowledge** due to the rise in the concept of **evidence-based practice** and secondly, health and social care professionals are increasingly **accountable** for the practice they deliver.

Critical thinking and the increase in professional knowledge

Many writers such as Moyer and Elliott (2004) have commented on the continual state of change in the modern world; the pace of change is so fast that what is published today may be out of date by the time you read it. This is just as true in health and social care as in any other setting. What you learn today in a lecture or in the workplace one day might be out of date tomorrow or indeed by the time you encounter a situation in which you put this new knowledge into practice. It is certainly true that *'change is happening all the time'* and we would argue that you should embrace change. One reason why there is constant change is that we are continuously acquiring new information about health and social care topics and this is mostly due to the increase in evidence-based practice.

What is evidence-based practice?

You may have heard of the term 'evidence-based practice'. Evidence-based practice is about being able to provide a strong rationale for your health or social care practice. Simply put:

> *evidence based practice is practice that is supported by clear reasoning, taking into account the patient's/client's preferences and using your own judgement.*
>
> (Aveyard and Sharp 2009: 7)

The importance of the concept of evidence-based practice is that it emphasizes the need for the best possible evidence to underpin practice. The concept of evidence-based practice has replaced the concept of practice based on tradition and ritual. Most definitions of evidence-based practice argue that in addition to evidence, professionals should use their professional judgement alongside consideration of patient or client preferences (Aveyard and Sharp 2009).

Information overload

Along with the rise in interest in evidence-based practice, there has been a vast increase in knowledge and evidence relating to professional practice. Some information is useful and some less useful. There is so much information available on any one health or social care topic that it can be difficult to read and comprehend everything related to your topic of study, let alone work out if the information is of good quality. This is why you need to be a critical thinker; so that you can work out what is useful information and what is less useful for your practice and academic writing.

Example

Writing in the *British Medical Journal* in 2010, Fraser and Dunstan cite the example of a cardiac surgeon who would need to read 40 papers each day, every day for 11 years to keep abreast of new developments in the field. Of course, at the end of these 11 years, these developments are already out of date!

This situation is roughly the same in every health and social care field. In addition to published academic papers, there are new websites, blogs and information resources for patients/clients. If you do a quick internet search using a search engine such as Google or Yahoo! on any health or social care topic, you will get many thousands of hits. This will be far too many to make any sense of. This is why you need a **more specific professional health or social care database** (which we will discuss in Chapter 3) rather than a general internet search engine when you are searching more seriously for health or social care topics. Using a more specific database will reduce the number of unwanted hits you get; however, you will still access many thousands of hits unless you are very focused in your search.

Let's take **for example** the topic of dementia, one that is potentially relevant to many health and social care professionals. CINAHL is the abbreviated title of a well-used database containing references for health and social care. A general search for information about dementia using this subject-specific database will yield you over 18,000 hits. If you are more specific and request only **research papers** about dementia, you will still get a few thousand hits. Reducing this further to a **particular aspect** of dementia care will reduce the number of hits further still, but they are still likely to run into many hundreds or a few thousand. Clearly this is a daunting number but it illustrates the point we are trying to make – the more focused your search is, the more you can narrow down your search and reduce the number of unwanted hits you get.

Consider one area of your professional or clinical practice (it may be a patient/client problem or intervention). Enter the key phrase into a database or search engine and see how many results (hits) you get. How do you think this would compare with 10 or 20 years ago?

You can see that if you are going to use evidence in your professional practice and academic writing you need to seek out the best available information for your studies and practice. You also need to focus on the specific aspect of the topic you are interested in so that you do not get sidetracked with more general information and therefore fail to find out what you really need to know. You also need to be selective about what you read, see and hear and be able to recognize good quality evidence when you come across it. It is important to make sense of what you read, see and hear so that you can work out what information is good quality and should influence your practice, and what isn't and should not. In general, **research** will be stronger evidence than more **anecdotal** sources and **reviews of research** will be stronger still. We will discuss these in more detail in Chapter 3.

Smith (2010) describes the responses from some health and social care workers to managing vast amounts of information. He points to the 'ostrich strategy' that is adopted by those who do not try to keep up to date, and the 'pigeon strategy' in which professionals 'cherry pick' what they want to believe from all the available information. This might include listening only to what they hear from colleagues in practice and not finding out more from a range of sources. In this book we argue that it is not good practice to accept the first thing you read, see or are told in practice without further investigation. You need to be more critical than this.

Professional knowledge is changing and expanding all the time. It is not possible to teach everyone how to respond in every given situation. As knowledge is increasing at such a fast pace, all students/learners and practitioners need to be confident in accessing new knowledge, and they need to be able to think critically about it. Professionals need skills to access and interpret the knowledge they require when they require it. We will not survive in professional life if we just try and remember facts or learn from experience, as we will quickly become out of date. Not only that, but we will then be role-modelling out of date practice for others to learn from. It doesn't take much imagination to see how practice can quickly become outdated if people learn from others who are not up to date. We need to be able to continue to keep up to date, and respond flexibly and creatively to solve problems in fast-changing health and social care environments.

In response to this information overload, the best strategy is not only to keep reading and accessing up-to-date information but also to be critical of the information you read so that you know which information is useful to you and which is less useful. The aim of this book is to show you how to do this most effectively.

It is not appropriate in the world of health and social care to accept everything you are told by lecturers and practice assessor/mentors or to learn just by observing role models and building up experience. You also need to:

- *Read widely about your topic and appraise the quality of what you are reading.*
- *Think critically about what you see and hear in practice.*
- *Think critically about how you seek out and use good quality information from a variety of sources.*
- *Think critically about how the best new evidence can be applied to your practice.*

Professional accountability

As a health or social care professional or student/learner you have a representative professional governing body. All of the professional bodies emphasize the importance of professional accountability for practice. As a practitioner, you must be able to justify and give a clear account of and rationale for your practice (Dimond 2008). According to Griffiths and Tengnah (2008), to be accountable is to be answerable for your acts and your omissions. This involves a duty to provide the most up-to-date care, based on the best available evidence. It is the role of the professional to incorporate relevant information into everyday practice in order to provide *safe and effective* patient/client care and to ensure that the best care is delivered. A key component of accountability is using evidence-based practice as a justification for the care or practice you give.

 *One reason it is so important to make sense of the information you come across is because as a health or social care professional, you are **accountable** for the care you give.*

The complicated part comes when you consider that most aspects of care are informed by a wealth of information – recent developments, research, policy documents, standards of practice and so on. For any one aspect of care that you consider, there is a vast amount of related literature. Not only is there a lot of reading to do, you also need to be critical of what you read and you need to make a judgement about it if you are to be able to account for your care or practice if called to do so.

Who are you accountable to?

- Students are accountable to their higher education institution, and when they are in practice settings they should be supervised by a registered professional.
- Registered practitioners are accountable to their professional body and their employers.
- All registered health and social care practitioners are accountable to the law.

Different professional bodies

In the United Kingdom, the **Health Professions Council** (HPC) currently regulates 15 professional groups (at the time of writing) including occupational therapists, physiotherapists, operating department practitioners, dieticians, paramedics, radiographers, speech and language therapists, art therapists, chiropodists/podiatrists, clinical scientists, orthoptists, prosthetists and orthotists. Their *Standards of Conduct, Performance and Ethics* (HPC 2008) are available at www.hpc-uk.org/aboutregistration/standards.

There are plans to transfer the General Social Care Council (GSCC) functions to the HPC in 2012 but currently social workers have a *Code of Practice for Employers of Social Care Workers* (GSCC 2010), available at www.gscc.org.uk/page/35/Codes+of+practice.html.

All branches of nursing and midwifery are accountable to the **Nursing and Midwifery Council** (NMC) which publishes *The Code: Standards of Conduct, Performance and Ethics for Nurses and Midwives* (NMC 2008), available at www.nmc-uk.org/Nurses-and-midwives/The-code.

All these professional organizations emphasize that those accountable to them should:

- Provide a high standard of practice at all times.
- Provide care that is based on the best available evidence.

Access your professional body's standards or code of conduct, performance and ethics. See if you can identify any parts of it which require you to be a critical thinker.

When you are called to account for your practice, you will only be able to do so if you have administered care that you can justify. It is no good trying to defend yourself by saying 'my colleague advised me to do this' or 'my lecturer told me to do this'. This will not be seen as a good justification for your actions, and would certainly not be seen as a strong defence. It is not difficult to see where these points are taking us. There is an ever increasing amount of information available for health and social care professionals to make sense of, and each professional has an obligation to make decisions based on the best available evidence in order to provide optimum care and remain accountable to their professional body. The best way to defend your practice is to provide appropriate evidence to justify your actions – you need to be able to think critically to be able to do this.

What about your legal responsibilities?

All professionals owe a legal duty of care to those they look after and this duty involves delivering care that is based on the best available evidence. Recent case law has supported the role of evidence, and using the best available evidence, to determine the standard of care professionals have to deliver rather than allowing professionals to disregard evidence and set their own standards.

However, this has been the case only recently. Not many years ago, the standard of care was largely set by professionals. This norm was established in a case frequently referred to as the Bolam case (*Bolam* v. *Friern Hospital Management Committee* [1957] 2 All ER 118 per McNair J.). This case focused on the care of a patient who was given electro-convulsive therapy (ECT) without the administration of muscle relaxant. He sustained an injury which he claimed was due to the failure to administer the muscle relaxant and the court considered whether there had been a breach of duty when the doctor decided not to administer the relaxant. In other words, did the doctor owe a duty to the patient to administer the relaxant? In order to answer this question, the court referred to other psychiatrists to see what the common practice was in respect of the administration of muscle relaxant. Because the court was informed that other psychiatrists would not have given the muscle relaxant, it ruled that this was not an essential practice and the patient lost his case. Thus at the time, the standard of care was set by the opinion of professional groups who did not have to rely on evidence to defend their practice. It was enough that other professionals would back them up, irrespective of what the evidence advised was best practice. This was known as the 'Bolam principle'.

You can see that the 'Bolam principle' did not demand that practice was evidence based; it only demanded that it was in accordance with what other professionals would do. Gradually this principle has been replaced by a requirement for professionals to be able to justify their actions with reference to evidence. In the case of *Bolitho* v. *City & Hackney Health Authority* [1993] 13 BMLR 111, CA, the court held that the body of expert opinion relied upon to judge good practice should be logical and evidence based, thus establishing a legal duty to provide care that is based on the best available evidence, rather than a repetition of other professionals' action or advice.

How critical thinking can help you in your academic assignments and professional decision-making

We have illustrated how we are often inundated with information, but a lot of it is poor quality and we therefore need to think critically about the information we are presented with. We have also illustrated with **Example 1** and **Example 2** earlier in this chapter that it is easy for a critical approach to be lost within a 'good story'. If this is considered to be unfortunate within everyday life, it is far worse and potentially far more serious within health and social care practice as professionals risk making poor decisions if they are not critical about the information upon which they base their practice. You can see how critical thinking is a skill that is essential to acquire and one which will enhance your academic writing and practice. We have illustrated this in **Example 3**.

If you examine the marking criteria for your academic assignments, you will see that you are marked on your ability to demonstrate that you can be critical of the literature you include. This involves using the best available evidence relating to the points you are making. In principle this generally means looking for research evidence rather than anecdotal sources. We also have to be aware of what constitutes good quality research and if at all possible look for reviews of research rather than single papers. It is also necessary to make a judgement about the quality of the research, which we will explain in later chapters. In your professional practice, this means questioning what you are told and looking up information to inform your care. Taking information at face value and out of context – even if it is published in a reputable professional journal – is not the way to attain academic or professional credibility.

The need for health and social care professionals to keep up to date with information regarding new developments and appraise the merits of new research and proposals in relation to their own practice is one of the main drivers behind the current move towards an 'all graduate' health and social care professional body and specialist and advanced roles. The need to be able to think critically as a safe, effective and independent practitioner has never been greater. It is likely that qualified professionals will be those who assess the patient/client and plan evidence-based care which may then be implemented by assistant practitioners, care assistants and those in supportive roles. As professionals we need to be critical thinkers in order to plan and evaluate the effectiveness of the interventions we deliver rather than carrying out care unquestioningly.

Before you move on to the rest of the book, can you identify how you might become more critical?

Because there is so much information available, in this book we make a distinction between information that is readily available – **for example**, lecture notes, recommended textbooks (which we discuss in Chapter 2) – and information for which you need to search a bit harder – **for example**, through a literature search to locate relevant journal articles (which we discuss in Chapter 3).

It is important to note that we will be discussing critical thinking in relation to both your academic studies *and* your professional practice. This is because practice and theory are closely interconnected. Sometimes you may be writing about what you have done in your workplace, or you may be applying knowledge or research gained from writing in relation to your management of care for a patient/client. It is hoped that this book will assist you in developing your skills as a critical thinker within health and social care. Read on . . .

In summary

We have discussed why it is important to be a critical thinker as this helps us to make rational decisions in our professional lives. We need to examine our own beliefs in order to do this and then think critically about the information we come across. There is a vast amount of literature and other information that you will encounter and you will need to make sense of what you read and not accept arguments at face value. We have suggested an approach to being critical of what you read, see or hear using the 'six questions to trigger critical thinking' given earlier. As a professional, you are accountable and you should ensure that the practice you deliver is evidence based. Critical thinking helps us to work out which evidence to use.

Key points

1 Critical thinking is essential to promote reasonable decision-making.
2 Critical thinking means being critical about the information we receive and how we use it.
3 Information is expanding in all areas of health and social care – some information is useful and relevant, some less so, and some can be inaccurate or misleading.
4 As professionals we need to be able to work out which information is useful to us and use it appropriately.
5 We suggest using the 'six questions to trigger critical thinking' approach to do this – this should help you to identify the most appropriate sources and enable you to be more critical of the information you use in your academic work and professional practice.

2

How you can think more critically about information that is readily available

What type of information is readily available? • Thinking critically about the quality and usefulness of 'readily available information' • In summary • Key points

In this chapter we will:

- Identify what is readily available information.
- Discuss how to judge the quality and usefulness of this information.
- Show how you can begin to think critically about the information you find and how to use it.

What type of information is readily available?

In this chapter we will look at the information that you will encounter on a day-to-day basis and we will refer to this as **'readily available information'**. By this we mean information that you do not have to search long and hard to find; you may just encounter it in your day-to-day professional or student life. There is so much of this information that it is important to be able to make sense of it and to know when it is of good enough quality upon which to base your professional practice or use in your academic work, and when you need to dig a bit deeper.

Think quickly and jot down all the places/people from which you currently get your information related to your studies and/or your practice.

Such forms of 'readily available information' may include:

- Newspapers and other forms of media.
- Websites focusing on health and social care.
- Internet search engines such as Google and Yahoo!.
- Lectures and lecture notes.
- Lecturers or practice assessor/mentors.
- Colleagues in your professional practice area.
- Textbooks.
- Journals to which your workplace/learning institution has a subscription.
- Professional policies and guidelines.
- Information leaflets by patient or client organizations.

It is also important to note that patients or clients are also frequently in receipt of this type of information and they may use the internet to find additional sources of information and a second opinion about their treatment. There are some well advertised and readily available sources where the public can seek information, either in the form of information leaflets produced by professional organizations or via the internet – **for example**:

- The British Broadcasting Corporation (BBC) health news at www.bbc. co.uk/news/health.
- Citizens Advice for a wider range of issues at www.citizensadvice.org.uk.
- Organizations that are targeted at the public such as Patient.co.uk at www. patient.co.uk/ or NHS Direct at www.nhsdirect.nhs.uk.

The problem with 'readily available information' is that there is so much of it around. This is partly a result of the information revolution and the free publication of ideas on the internet. Anyone can publish anything online and you need to be a critical reader to work out whether what you are reading is a reliable source of information. **For example**, anyone can add or edit information on Wikipedia (http://en.wikipedia.org/wiki) so you cannot be sure whether information about health and social care issues has been submitted by a reliable or knowledgeable source.

Thinking critically about the quality and usefulness of 'readily available information'

Let's have a look at some of the sources of 'readily available information' and work out whether they are reliable enough for you to use in your professional practice and academic writing. Remember to use the '**six questions to trigger critical thinking**' to work out the strengths and weaknesses of the information you have.

Newspapers

In Chapter 1, we gave an example of how newspapers can use misleading statistics to promote a story. This should be enough of a warning against using media information in your academic work or any practice situation without seeking further information. However, newspapers may provide useful background information. For example, they might lead you to a controversial quotation to start your assignment or to get people thinking in a discussion. Or they might refer you to a research study, giving a snippet of information but not the full reference for the study, making it harder (but possible) to track it down. In principle, you should avoid direct reference to newspaper articles in your written work or discussions at work unless you use them as a springboard for further enquiry or you are discussing the media's view or perspective on a topic. Some newspapers may have stricter editorial quality control than others and so may offer a higher standard of information but this still needs to be checked out.

Internet sources

The World Wide Web contains many hundreds of millions of pages of information, including everything from rigorous research to trivia and misinformation. Useful websites are likely to be those that are produced by a recognized professional body or patient/client group. These might contain guidelines for practice, up-to-date news on professional issues and issues of concern to patient and client groups. You will also find blogs and professional opinion which may offer really up-to-date and rapidly changing information.

Sometimes you can access academic journal articles on the internet from a simple search using a search engine such as Google or Yahoo!. However, unless you use an appropriate search strategy, as discussed in the next chapter, you are unlikely to get a good range of relevant research from a random internet search.

How can you judge the quality of a website?

Before making use of information found on the web in your academic work or practice, you need to make sure it is high quality and up to date. Remember to use the 'six questions to trigger critical thinking' given in Chapter 1, for example:

- **What is the evidence that is reported?** If a website refers to the conclusion of a piece of research, remember that you should try and access the *original* research if you are using this in your assignments or practice.
- **Who has written the website?** Consider whether the author is a credible expert on the topic and if they are likely to have a bias or 'hidden agenda' on the topic – **for example**, are they from a campaign group trying to get a particular drug or vaccination banned (consider the publicity surrounding the MMR vaccination mentioned in the previous chapter).
- **When was the site produced?** Do not assume it is up to date just because it is still on the internet. See if you can locate the date it was written.
- **Who is the target audience?** Remember to use the information in this context. It may be pitched for patients/clients rather than for professionals.

In general, if you refer to a website in your academic work, you must assess the quality of the site and whenever possible you should go to the original sources it has cited. Consider whether it is the best evidence you can find or whether you should just use it as a springboard for further debate. Citing websites, like newspapers, without judging their quality, is like telling the marker, *'I was in a bit of a rush and this is all I could find . . .'* and your mark will undoubtedly reflect this. Similarly, if you go to your professional practice area with only a website as a recommendation for change, you will probably be encouraged to find stronger evidence. Remember that if you use information from the web, the relevant web page(s) must be fully cited in your reference list as it is needed for any academic work or publication you refer to. You may wish to check whether your organization or university has a guide to referencing web pages.

Advice from practice assessors/mentors and colleagues

Practice assessors/mentors and colleagues are an obvious source of professional knowledge and an obvious means by which that knowledge can be passed on from one person to another. Such people are, and have always been, a valuable resource. Indeed many studies suggest that professional decisions are often made relying on advice passed on from one colleague to another, rather than seeking information from other sources. Research also suggests that the information passed between colleagues is valued and often remembered for years and years to come (Gabbay and Le May 2004; Turner and Whitfield 2006). We all learn a lot from role-modelling from other professionals and most of us can remember a good role model. Indeed, learning from other professionals is a major part of professional education. However, you need to remember that health and social care providers are a wide and diverse group. There are expert practitioners and there are novice practitioners. There are practitioners who are thoughtful and reflective about their practice and there are those who are not. The quality of advice you receive in practice may vary!

How can you judge if information from practice assessors, mentors or colleague is of good quality?

If a practice assessor/mentor or colleague tells you something about an intervention or care decision, consider the '**six questions to trigger critical thinking**'. **For example**, consider whether they are quoting from their own experience or from research evidence or guidelines. Where there is no research evidence relating to a complex and unusual problem then experience and reflective judgement can be very valuable. But you need to decide if it is the best available evidence, and you should 'check it out' for accuracy.

Discussion between professionals about information or research that has been critically appraised is likely to be beneficial. However, it is not always the case that information will be critically appraised by practitioners. Referring back to our discussion of the need to be critical of what you read, see and hear, you therefore need to question what you are told in practice rather than accepting what your practice assessor/mentor or colleague tells or shows you. The examples of the reporting of the Implanon story (**Example 1**, Chapter 1) and the MMR vaccination story (**Example 2**, Chapter 1) show how misinformation can easily spread when information is not critically appraised. If you stop to think about this, the implications are enormous. If information or advice is not critically appraised or is based on unfounded rumour, and is then passed unchallenged from one professional to another, we will not be demonstrating evidence-based practice and we will certainly not be applying critical thinking! So beware of accepting information at face value from your practice assessor/mentor and your colleagues. We will discuss this further in Chapter 5.

Lectures

Lectures may only provide a basic introduction to a topic. To gain a full understanding of the topic, you are expected to access the given references or reading list and read more broadly around the subject. We cannot stress enough how important it is do this! If you only refer to lecture notes in your assignment or use them as evidence for your practice it implies that you have not been thinking critically or in depth about the subject. It gives the same message as described previously: *'I was in a rush and did not have time to find evidence related to the lecture.'* You would therefore be unlikely to gain high marks in assignments or be able to give an adequate reason for your practice decisions. There is one exception to this, which is if you have a lecture from a leading authority or expert on a topic and he or she is delivering material that is as yet unpublished. Then, and only then, may you quote from this lecture in your assignment or discuss their ideas in practice without finding further supporting information. However, even then your argument will be stronger if you find related evidence to back up what you write.

How can you judge the quality of a lecture?

When you are in a lecture, consider the '**six questions to trigger critical thinking**'. Consider the sources that the lecturer is referring to and whether the arguments they present make sense. Our advice is that you should avoid referring *only* to a lecture in your written work or practice. Instead, use the ideas generated in the lecture, read up some of the references and refer to these instead. It is far better still to search more widely on the topic, as we will discuss in the next chapter – a lecture should be used as a **basis for further reading and investigation**.

Unfortunately a lot of people rely on information they have received in a lecture without doing the appropriate reading. They also rely on this information for years to come. The implications of this are similar to what happens if practice information is passed from one colleague to another without critical thinking. We quickly become out of date. If we are to become independent critical thinkers we need to move on from this approach and use lectures as they are meant to be used – as launch-pads for further reading and discussion.

Textbooks

Textbooks, especially at undergraduate level, generally provide a springboard for further study. Some textbooks provide a basic overview of current knowledge on a particular area, especially if you are starting out in a topic. They may provide sound factual information on topics such as anatomy and physiology. Others provide ideas, theoretical models and frameworks or opinions on a topic by leading experts. The main thing is to ensure that you have identified the most appropriate textbook for your purpose.

How do you know if a textbook is a useful one?

Consider the '**six questions to trigger critical thinking**'. Consider who the author is, the date of publication and the target audience. Be prepared to use the textbook as a springboard for further reading.

We suggest you do not start with a specialist book if you are new to a topic. This is because when you are starting to study a topic, it is usually most helpful to have an overview of the topic rather than to start by focusing on a specialist area which you may not be able to put into context. Do use the information on the back cover to find out who the book is aimed at and what the contents cover. Consider whether the textbook is appropriate for your level and focus of study. We also suggest that you read the reviews of textbooks and follow recommendations on your reading lists for core texts, noting who these are aimed at. Remember that a book can take many months and sometimes years to get into print so consider how up to date the information is and whether there are likely to be changes in the evidence used to support the arguments given in the book. Finally, make sure that you have the most up-to-date edition of any textbook you use, remembering that new editions of most popular texts are generally published every few years. Look at the date of the references used in the book too. Those who mark your work will notice if you are referring to an older version of a recently updated book.

Hard copy or electronic journals

Many workplaces subscribe to a journal, either in a hardbound copy or using an online electronic journals facility. If you find this is the case in your work or practice area, try and find out why that particular journal was chosen. It may be a specialist journal that publishes all the best research in that topic area. Remember that information found in one journal will not usually give you the range and breadth of literature that is available on a particular topic. There will be different information available in other journals and you might not get the 'whole picture' if you refer to just one journal. Please refer to Chapter 3 where we discuss how to search for a wider range of literature.

One research paper, even if it is a piece of good quality research relevant to your topic, is rarely enough for you to base a judgement on regarding correct practice or an academic argument. For any one study supporting a view, there may be four other papers that have a contradictory view.

How can you judge the quality of what you find in a journal?

There is a wide variety of information in all types of journals – from editorials to original research papers, to letters to the editor. It is important that you can recognize the types of information you may come across and use this appropriately in your written work or practice environment.

When you apply the '**six questions to trigger critical thinking**', consider carefully the 'what' so that you are clear about the type of information you have – **for example**, is it an editorial, an actual research study (if so, what type?), a descriptive literature review or a systematic review, or an overview of the topic? These are explained below. One important thing to remember is that journals that are easily available in your workplace will not provide a comprehensive range of relevant information on a topic. A full range of relevant information may be published in a variety of other sources and you will only find these through carrying out a comprehensive search – we will discuss this in Chapter 3.

What information will you find in a journal?

Editorials

These are written by the editor of a journal and represent his or her viewpoint or the viewpoint of the editorial team.

Systematic reviews

These are reviews of research undertaken on a particular topic and are generally presented using a research structure, as described here. They should have:

- A question or statement of aims.
- Method (which should outline the approach to the search).
- Results or findings.
- Discussion.
- Conclusions.

They should discuss how the quality of the research was appraised. The most comprehensive collection of systematic reviews is from the Cochrane Collaboration. These are reviews compiled by expert 'systematic reviewers' and published on the Cochrane Collaboration website, www.cochrane.org.

Unsystematic reviews or descriptive reviews

These may give a broad overview of a topic drawing on a wide range of literature. However, unless the approach to finding the literature is thorough and there is a specific question and method for the search, you cannot be sure that all the evidence on the topic has been included and there may be some bias in the selection of studies used. You should also note whether the quality of the research used has been appraised. This type of review will provide weaker evidence than one which has been compiled systematically. However, that is not to say that the information will not be useful to you, as such reviews may provide a concise (but not comprehensive) introduction to, or overview of, a topic. If you refer to this type of review in your written work, make sure that you are clear about the type of evidence you are using.

Research studies

Research studies generally provide stronger evidence than more anecdotal sources. These can be identified as they normally begin with a specific **research question or aim** which is addressed using an identified **method**, following which the **results or findings**, **discussion** and **conclusions** are given. They can be quantitative or qualitative and there are various approaches that can be taken within these broad areas. Research studies can provide good sources of evidence but they still need to be appraised individually. Be wary of a single piece of research evidence that makes a claim about practice. Consider a jigsaw where you only have one bit of the picture; sometimes you cannot tell what the final view will be. Instead, as we will discuss in the next chapter, it is better to search more broadly for more research papers or to locate a systematic review that has already been carried out. This is so you can gain an overview of what the conclusion is from all the research on the topic – i.e. complete the whole jigsaw.

Discussion or opinion papers

These will not have as clear a structure as a research study and will be introduced as representing the opinion of the author. Remember that the quality of this type of evidence will depend on the expertise of the person writing the paper – do not assume that even an expert will be basing their argument on relevant and evidence-based sources. They may be also be biased – not necessarily intentionally – in the selection of the sources they use. – Our advice is that you should only use this type of evidence when you cannot find research evidence on your topic.

Professional and clinical guidance, policies and 'evidence based' knowledge summaries

The move towards providing summaries of evidence either in policy or guidelines, or as standalone publications, is one of the most useful developments in health and social care. You might see paper volumes or links to internet sites that summarize the best available evidence.

If you come across up-to-date policy or guidelines based on the evidence from systematic reviews or summaries of systematic reviews, you have strong evidence upon which to base your professional practice or academic work.

These publications are different from other types of 'readily accessible' information because they are based not only on research but on systematic reviews of research of best available evidence. Below we have listed some examples of these publications:

- **Evidence in Health and Social Care** launched in 2009, has a search facility and ranks research according to relevance and quality. See **www.evidence. nhs.uk/default.aspx.**
- **The National Library of Guidelines** is a collection of guidelines for the NHS. It is based on the guidelines produced by the National Institute for Health and Clinical Excellence (NICE – www.nice.org.uk) and other national agencies. NICE describes itself as 'an independent organization responsible for providing national guidance on promoting good health and preventing and treating ill health'. NICE issues guidelines considered to be of very high quality because they are based on a systematic review of the evidence and involve extensive consultation not only with clinicians but also with patients/clients and, where relevant, industry.
- **Map of Medicine** describes itself as providing 'health guides which show you the ideal, evidence-based patient/client journey for common and important conditions. It is a high-level overview that can be shared by patients/clients and healthcare providers'. Information is available at www.mapofmedicine.com/

How do you know if the guidelines or knowledge summaries are of high quality?

We argue that these guidelines or summaries of best available evidence are an extremely useful resource for your academic and professional practice and they are readily available, usually in the practice environment. So how can you tell which of these guidelines and summaries are of good quality? You can apply the '**Six questions to trigger critical thinking**' to guidelines that you use. There are also tools that have been developed for the evaluation of guidelines, such as AGREE, which is available at www.agreecollaboration.org/instrument, and a tool called DISCERN which is used to ascertain the quality of written information on treatment choices: www. discern.org.uk.

> Generally there should be a good explanation of how the guidelines or summaries were compiled. The sources that were used should be clearly identified; these should be from best available evidence, usually research and systematic reviews of research. You should also check if they are up to date and have a review date.

If you come across guidelines and policy that appear to be evidence based, then these are likely to be strong evidence. This is because guidelines and policy from reliable sources (as in the examples given above) are compiled from the evidence from systematic reviews. In other words, they have done the hard work of searching for the best available evidence (as we discuss in the next chapter).

Access one of the websites above and see if you can find some guidelines that are relevant to you in your professional role.

Remember . . .

You should 'think critically' about every source of information that you are considering using.

In summary

In this chapter we have outlined the readily available information that you may come across in your everyday life as a student/learner or as a professional. The range of readily available information is vast and it is important that you can judge the quality and relevance of what you find. We have argued that newspaper articles and news items as well as many websites can be misleading and that they should be referred to minimally. They should certainly not be used in the main body of your assignment or as the focus of decision-making within professional practice. Information from practice assessors/colleagues and from lecture notes should be used only as a springboard for further study, rather than as an end in itself. Textbooks and academic journals that you encounter 'at random' may or may not be the most appropriate for your academic and professional learning needs, so consider their use carefully. If you come across a useful article in a journal in your placement area, you need to consider what type of paper it is, and whether there are other articles that are also relevant which would add to or 'complete the picture' of evidence on that topic. If you find well developed and established guidelines – especially those produced nationally by an established organization, then you have come across some high quality evidence.

Remember that 'readily available information' is usually just the 'tip of the iceberg' of the total information available on a particular topic. In order to find a more comprehensive picture, you need to search more thoroughly, as we will discuss in the next chapter.

Key points

1 There is a vast amount of 'readily available' information around. Such *readily available* evidence generally represents the 'tip of the iceberg' of information available.
2 This ranges from information which can be inaccurate and misleading to useful sources.
3 Try to avoid referencing media sources or unevaluated websites in your assignments.
4 Use lecture notes and advice from practice assessors/mentors and colleagues as a springboard for further study.
5 Remember that books and articles found in journals need to be viewed alongside other relevant publications.
6 Professional guidelines and summaries of evidence generally provide strong evidence if they are up to date and based on best available evidence.

3

Being more critical: how you can find the 'best available' evidence

Why do you need to dig deeper to find evidence? • Beginning the search process • Using subject-specific electronic databases • How can you plan and search for literature using specific databases? • What is the 'best available' evidence? • Research evidence • In summary • Key points

In this chapter we will:

- Explain why you need to dig a little deeper to find the 'best available' evidence.
- Explore the value of using specific databases to search for evidence, and examine how to plan and search for evidence using specific databases.
- Discuss how to find the best available evidence.
- Discuss what type of research you should look for and how you know when you have found it.

Why do you need to dig deeper to find evidence?

You can see from the discussion in Chapter 2 that you need to think carefully about information that is 'readily available', make a judgement about its quality and decide if you need to dig a little deeper to find the best available evidence. It is then important to think critically and to question the information you find so that you can recognize the best available evidence when you come across it.

You need to try and ensure you get the whole picture rather than relying on just the first piece of 'readily available information' you find.

We argued in Chapter 2 that unless you come across guidelines or policies relating to your practice that are based on the best available evidence, then most information that is readily available (that is, information that you do not need to search too hard for) generally provides just the 'tip of the iceberg' of available information on a topic and is generally best used as a springboard for further investigation or study.

You need to dig deeper because:

- As a 'critical thinker' you should not just accept the most readily available information; instead, you need to adopt a questioning approach and search for all the available information.
- One piece of research on its own is generally not enough – other studies may provide a different view or when viewed together may lead you to a different overall conclusion.
- The quality of information on websites and in the media may vary and may be biased.
- You need to be certain that you have found all the most up-to-date sources of evidence.
- You should review all the evidence on your topic rather than just select evidence that agrees with your argument.
- There may be more up to date and more relevant evidence that has become recently available.

In other words, a systematic and thorough search will ensure that you have obtained all or most of the evidence on a topic. You can demonstrate to the marker of your assignment or your colleagues in practice that you have searched in a comprehensive way, showing that you have been thorough in your approach rather than just relying on readily available sources.

Beginning the search process

In most cases, the best way to search is through your academic library, either online via your library's electronic resources, or in person. Without doing this, you are unlikely to access the best available evidence on your topic. Even if you find relevant journal articles by looking at a recent edition of a journal, you need to remember that you are only accessing a tiny proportion of evidence that is available on that particular topic. You do not know about information that has been published previously. You need to make sure that you do not just 'cherry pick' evidence you want to include. You are demonstrating a **critical approach** when you decide to search more thoroughly for further evidence. This is because you recognize that the evidence you have obtained through readily accessible sources is likely to be insufficient for your purposes.

Why not use Google or other search engines?

*Internet search engines such as Google, Bing or Yahoo! are **not** specific enough to search effectively for evidence. Beware of using only sources retrieved through search engines. Their ability to search is limited and so the information you find may be too broad, of poor quality, or you may have missed a key piece of research.*

Most people are very familiar with general internet search engines such as Google, Bing or Yahoo!. We use them on an everyday basis to search for a wide variety of things. However, they are not specific enough to find the best available professional evidence because they do not distinguish between what is good evidence and what is not. They simply present you with a list of hits and because there is so much information available to you it is very difficult, if not impossible, to identify what is worth looking at in more depth from all the hits you get.

For this reason, for your academic and professional searches you need a search engine which is subject-specific and which does not trawl through all the 'lay' publications and other sources of information that relate to your topic. Having said that, doing a quick search using an internet search engine such as Google on a topic you wish to explore further might give you some ideas of the terms or language used around your topic. So it might be worth a 'quick look' just to see what words you can then use to search using the more specific professional databases. A slightly more focused search can be carried out on Google Scholar (selected from the 'more' drop-down menu, where you can select type of publication and dates). However this would still not be a comprehensive search.

Think about how many hits you get (and how many of them are completely irrelevant) when you use Google or another search engine to look for something in your everyday life outside work. You can see why it is best not to use such search engines for your professional needs.

Using subject-specific electronic databases

In order to take a critical approach to your academic writing and professional practice, you can see that you need to be comprehensive and organized in your search for appropriate evidence. The best way to do this is by using a **subject-specific database**.

Why should you use a subject-specific database, instead of using a more casual approach to finding literature?

- You will find a broader range of literature relevant to your topic (**breadth**).
- You are more likely to find appropriate literature (**relevance**).
- You are more likely to find literature of good quality (**rigour**).
- Your search will be more comprehensive (**thoroughness**).

What is a subject-specific database?

Subject-specific databases hold the references for, and often abstracts or the full text version of, journal articles and many other texts, for which you can search using key words. There are many subject-specific databases which are each related to a particular academic field or professional group(s), **for example** health and/or social care. They are usually best accessed through your academic or professional library website. A database is simply a way of storing, organizing, searching and accessing information. It is a bit like a large electronic filing cabinet.

How do you find a subject-specific database?

If you go to the website of your academic or professional library or contact your subject librarian, you will usually find a list of databases which are relevant to your field of professional practice. Each database will have a description of its scope and focus, **for example**, some are psychology related, some are social science based, some are medically focused while others focus on literature for allied health care professionals – and so on. This is where you need to be thinking creatively and critically in terms of deciding what focus you are looking for. **For example**, you need to consider whether information from other professions may add insight and whether you have considered a holistic approach to your issue (e.g. you could consider psychological, cultural or educational issues that may require using a different database). If you are not sure which database to access, ask someone at your local university or from your professional development team.

You can see that you might use more than one database if you are doing a very thorough search. If you are not confident using computers then you may find it easier to visit the library in person and access training courses on how to search using databases. One thing to remember is that these databases do change their format or their names on a fairly regular basis. If you are returning to searching after a break, do check with your subject librarian which database is best for your needs. Also, remember that different databases operate slightly differently so do consult the information provided with the database to ensure that you make full use of the searching facility.

Key words and phrases

When you access a database you will be invited to enter a key word. You will then be invited to refine your search using that key word: by date, type of evidence, whether the key word appears in the whole text or just the abstract, and so on. If you widen the search and ask for all entries that have the key word in the whole text you are likely to be inundated with references. If you are more selective – **for example**, by requesting keyword entries from paper abstracts only – you will limit your search.

How can you plan and search for literature using specific databases?

The process of searching for literature is discussed in detail in the partner book in this series, *A Beginner's Guide to Evidence Based Practice* by Aveyard and Sharp (2009). In this book we discuss using the acronym PICOT to help you identify what you are trying to find out. Each letter prompts you to consider a different aspect of the situation you are seeking information about:

Population
Intervention or issue

Comparison or context
Outcome
Time

(Stillwell *et al.* 2010)

- **Population:** we need to consider who are the people we are interested in investigating with similar characteristics such as gender, age, condition, problem, location, role, **for example**, older people in residential care, those who are homeless, mothers under 45, patient/clients who have had knee replacements, patient/clients who have accessed paramedic services for chest pain, staff who work out of hours, students who access study advice and so on.
- **Intervention/issue:** these can be diagnostic, therapeutic, preventative, exposure, managerial, experiences, perceptions, costs, etc.
- **Comparisons/context:** this can be against another intervention or no intervention. Comparisons can be made against national or professional standards or guidelines. The context of the study can be where the study takes place.
- **Outcome:** faster, cheaper, reduction or increase in symptoms, events, episodes, prognosis, mortality, accuracy, etc.
- **Time:** this may or may not be relevant, for example, days post-op or post-intervention, within 24 hours of accessing the service, etc.

Identifying what you need to find out

- Think carefully about what you want to find out (consider the PICOT prompt, or maybe make a spider diagram or list all of the issues).
- Identify your key words and use a thesaurus to find alternative words (synonyms).
- Set limits on the search requested – consider whether you want to limit the number of hits you get by specifying language, date, title or abstract.
- Use Boolean operators as discussed below.
- Find out how each database operates, bearing in mind that they are all slightly different.

- **Keywords** should reflect the topic you are searching for, remembering to use all words, not just those currently in use. Think widely and laterally!
- **Boolean operators** help you refine the search . . .
  - **AND** ensures that **each term** you have entered is searched for. This will reduce the number of hits you get as each term must be included in the article for it to be recognized . . .
  - **OR** ensures that **either one term or another** is selected. This will increase the number of hits you get as you only need to identify one of the terms for the article to be selected.

- There is also the * facility (on some databases this is another symbol – do check!) which enables you to identify all possible endings of the key term you write. To use this, you need to identify the 'root' of the word – i.e. the part of the word that doesn't change – and put the * after that last letter. **For example**: Disab* will find you **disability, disabl**ed and **disabilities.**

Planning your search

The following key word search table (Aveyard and Sharp 2009) illustrates how you could to plan your search using truncated words, and the AND/OR facility.

	1		2		3
a)	Disab* or		Attitud*or		Student*or
b)	Handicap*or		Belief *or		Learner* or
c)	Or		Valu* or		or
d)	Or	AND	Mindset* or	AND	or
e)			Approach*		

Set your limits

You can also specify whether you would like to search throughout **the whole article** for the term, or whether you are going to limit your search to the **abstract** or **title**.

- If you limit your search to the identification of the term in just the title, you will exclude a lot of references which might be relevant to you, even though the title does not use the key terms you have identified.
- Conversely, if you search through all the articles for your key word, you may be overwhelmed with literature.

You should therefore consider selecting the abstract as this gives a brief overview of what the article contains and what type of writing it is.

Documenting your search strategy

It is helpful in all your assignments if you can document *how* you searched for the best available evidence rather than just relying on readily available information. This demonstrates that you took a critical approach to finding your evidence and did not use the first pieces of information that came to hand. We have developed the following chart which enables you to do this.

Database (use one row for each database)	Limitations set	Key search terms (include truncation, wildcard and Boolean operators, or medical subject/thesaurus headings used)	Number of hits
Example Cinahl	1990–2011, English language only, word appearing in abstract only	female OR women OR woman AND catheter	251

Remember . . .

- Searching for literature is time consuming and is a skill that needs to be developed over time – you are advised not to leave it until the last minute.
- If you do not have any 'hits' from your search, then keep searching with different key words, or you may need to broaden your topic until you identify literature which is linked to your subject area.
- If you have too many hits, you will need to re-focus your search, maybe by date or language.
- You need to keep a record of the search terms you have used and the results of these searches, and include these in your assignment, perhaps in an appendix.
- Even if you do not find any evidence, this is still a useful 'finding' as long as you can demonstrate that your search has been thorough.

How to find additional evidence that may not be found using databases

Electronic searches of subject-specific databases are not 100 per cent comprehensive and are unlikely to identify all the relevant literature on your topic.

Despite the advances in technology, electronic searching is not 100 per cent effective or accurate. This means that you can miss key evidence through electronic searching. The reasons for this are as follows:

- Some relevant literature might have been categorized using different key words and would therefore not be identified by one particular searching strategy.

- The topic you are looking for may only be briefly mentioned in papers discussing broader topics and therefore is not identified by key words or in the index when these papers are entered onto the database. As a result, they may not be recognized when you search.
- The title of the paper may be misleading, **for example** some authors use humorous titles or phrases that you may not be familiar with.

If you want to be really thorough, additional approaches to take when searching for evidence are:

- Look in the reference lists of the papers you *have* found (this process is called snowballing).
- Look through the contents pages of back copies of journals which you have previously found useful.
- Ask experts who may have attended conferences or who have access to as yet unpublished ideas or contacts.
- Supplement your search with the more readily available literature, as identified in Chapter 2.
- Search for papers written by experts in the field.

Remember, though, that this type of searching is an 'add on' to your electronic search rather than a substitute.

Getting hold of your sources

The references to which you are directed are likely to be found in journals, books and other publications. Books are generally held in a library and you will need to access these in person; however, the number of books available electronically in the form of e-books is growing in many library facilities. Do check with your academic or professional librarian for further information about this.

Journals can generally be accessed either in person from the library where they are held as hard copies, or online though a library's electronic journals collection. You are strongly advised to become familiar with your electronic library as most university and workplace libraries will have many journals accessible in **'full-text'** format electronically so that you can locate and download many articles without leaving your computer. **You will need a password to access these.** There is sometimes – but not always – a link from the search engine database to the full text article in the electronic library.

Using abstracts to select the most useful results

Once you have completed a search, you need to work out what type of evidence you have identified on your chosen topic. Depending on the number of hits you have, you probably cannot download or access all of it and you need to make sense of what you have found. It is better not to rely on the title alone as this can be misleading. This is because the focus of the article is often unclear from the title alone. Instead read the abstract.

An **abstract** is a short summary of what the paper is about which is usually printed before the beginning of the paper. It is often available directly through the subject-specific database even if access to the full article is not. The abstract will give you a summary of the content of the article, in particular stating whether or not it is a research article.

See if you can find several different journal papers and look at their abstracts. See if you can tell what type of paper each one is (e.g. a review, research or opinion).

What is the 'best available' evidence?

Once you have found your evidence you need to consider what type of evidence is most useful to you. In other words, what exactly should you be looking for? You may have heard of the term '**hierarchy of evidence**'. Strong evidence is at the top of the hierarchy and weaker evidence is at the bottom. Classifications as to what counts as strong evidence vary according to what you are trying to find out as we will see in the examples later on in this chapter.

In general terms, you will find the **literature review**, in particular the **systematic review** at the top of the hierarchy of evidence in almost every classification you will come across. The systematic review is generally considered to be the most useful information you can find. A systematic review is a very detailed literature review and seeks to summarize all available evidence on a topic. Less detailed reviews are called literature reviews.

If you come across a systematic review when you search for evidence then you have probably found the best available evidence for your topic, especially if the review is recent and it is clear that it has been carried out thoroughly. You can probably stop searching and use this review to inform your practice and academic work. Less detailed reviews will also be useful to you.

How can you recognize a literature review when you see one?

Authors of a review have not done their own first-hand study (e.g. experiments or interviews) but instead have collected together the research of others in order to reach a new conclusion. Good reviews will tell you how they have been undertaken; they are usually set out in the same way as a research paper. A good systematic literature review will be written up in the same manner as a research article, with a **research or review question, aims** and objectives and a methods section outlining how the review was under-taken. The method should tell you how the researchers searched for literature, what literature they included and why, and what they excluded and why. By reading the method, you should have a good idea about how the researchers carried out their literature review. The conclusion is based on weighing up all the literature on the topic area. You may find that that a review concludes that the research evidence is consistent in its findings or that there is insufficient high-quality evidence. This is just as important to informing professional practice and our writing as a strong positive or negative result from research.

Systematic reviews

A systematic review is the most detailed type of review and aims to identify and track down *all* the available literature on a topic with clear explanations of the approach taken (methodology). Systematic literature reviews are referred to as original empirical research as they review primary data, which can be either quantitative or qualitative.

Systematic reviews which have a detailed research methodology should be regarded as a strong form of evidence when they are identified as relevant to a literature review question.

The most well known method for conducting a systematic review is produced by the **Cochrane Collaboration**. See the Cochrane website where you can browse by topic for reviews and they have a plain English summary to help you understand complex jargon. Information about the Cochrane Library reviews is available at www.cochrane.org/reviews.

A systematic review undertaken in the detail required by the Cochrane Collaboration is usually considered to be the most detailed and robust form of review that exists. **For example**, in the UK they are used in the formulation of guidelines for NICE, available at http://www.nice.org.uk. NICE recommendations for clinical practice are based on the best available evidence. Alternatively, the Centre for Reviews and Dissemination is a useful and reliable source and has a database relating to health policy and practice: www.york.ac.uk/inst/crd.

For social policy and social care, see the website of the Social Care Institute for Excellence (SCIE)at www.scie.org.uk/research/reviews.asp or The University of York web page on Systematic Reviews in Social Policy and Social Care at www.york.ac.uk/inst/chp/srspsc/publications.htm.

Why are systematic reviews so useful?

Literature reviews are important because they seek to:

- Summarize all the literature that is available on any one topic.

- Prevent one 'high profile' piece of information having too much influence.
- Present an analysis of the available literature so that the reader does not have to access each individual research report included in the review.

Before you carry out any database searches, access one of the websites above that contain systematic reviews and you may save yourself hours of searching other databases.

Descriptive (or narrative) literature reviews

A literature review can be approached in a systematic manner even if the detail required by the Cochrane Collaboration is not attained. However, as stated above, you should find a section in the study in which the method of undertaking the review is outlined. This then enables you to judge the quality of the review. You should read the method by which the review has been carried out to see how rigorously the review has been undertaken. Beware of reviews which do not have a published method telling the reader how the review has been carried out or where this is only briefly described. These are sometimes referred to as **narrative** or **descriptive reviews**. This type of review might be no more than a biased or randomly assembled collection of research papers about a given topic. Consequently, the conclusions drawn are likely to be inaccurate.

Although it may refer to a lot of literature or evidence, a narrative literature review does not tell you how the authors identified or why they included this literature. You do not know if the writers just 'cherry picked' the literature they wanted to include, ignoring everything else. Many, many papers in health and social care are written in this way. While you might find them useful for information, you should be aware that they do not necessarily give you a comprehensive range of information on the topic because they do not tell you the criteria by which they included information. If you find an information or discussion article which has included various references and wonder if it is a literature review, have a look to see if there is a clearly written methods section telling you how the information included was identified. If no such methods section exists then the article is not strictly a 'literature review' – or at least not a detailed one – instead, it is more likely to be an informative discussion of literature.

What if you cannot find a literature review or systematic review?

If no reviews are available, the next best thing is to access individual pieces of research on a topic. If you have done a thorough and focused search, you will see the range of research papers that are available on your topic, rather than just identifying one paper as you might if you just flick through a journal that you come across. It is important to remember that one individual piece of research – however good it is – is never enough evidence on its own to recommend a change in practice. Therefore if you cannot find a review, then look at as many research articles as you can on the topic you are interested in. In the absence of a review, these will be your best available evidence.

Research evidence

Recognizing research papers

You can recognize a research paper from a 'non research' paper by the way that it is structured. As with a literature review, a research paper will have a **research question, stated aims** and a **methods** section which tells you how the research was undertaken. There follows a **results** or **findings** section and a **discussion** with **recommendations**.

What type of individual research papers should you look for?

In very general terms, research is divided into two types:

- **Qualitative.**
- **Quantitative.**

It is very useful to consider what type of research will address what you are hoping to find out (this does not matter as much in a literature review as reviews can contain both qualitative and quantitative papers). When there is no literature review, you need to think about the type of research that is most useful to you. The type of research you find is often determined by the type of question you are asking. So you need to **think critically** about this before you start your search. First of all it is useful to consider the main differences between qualitative and quantitative research.

The main differences between qualitative and quantitative research

Qualitative research generally uses interviews to explore the **experience** or meaning of an issue in depth. The results are presented as **words**.

Quantitative research generally explores if something is **effective** or not, or measures the **amount** of something. Results are generally presented using **numbers** or statistics.

What is the best type of research to look for after a literature review?

Some topics are best explored using qualitative research and others will be best explored using quantitative research. Therefore it is not possible to say which type of research is better in any general sense. There is broad agreement that literature reviews are at the top of the hierarchy of evidence for all situations you can think of. After that, it depends on what you are looking for. You may come across the so-called traditional 'hierarchy of evidence'. This hierarchy applies to situations only when you need to measure the effectiveness of something; **for example**, does something work or not?

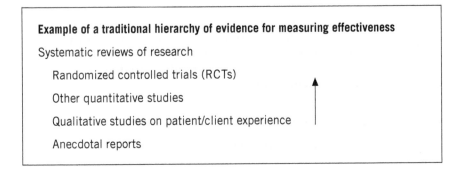

Example of a traditional hierarchy of evidence for measuring effectiveness

Systematic reviews of research

    Randomized controlled trials (RCTs)

    Other quantitative studies

    Qualitative studies on patient/client experience

    Anecdotal reports

Do not be misled into thinking that this hierarchy works for all situations. **If only things were so simple!** There is a danger of oversimplification here. Unfortunately there is not one hierarchy that works for all situations. While it is probably true that a systematic review will be most useful to you, after that what is most useful depends on what you are hoping to find out. Different situations require different types of evidence. You can see from the discussion of qualitative and quantitative research above that the two approaches are different and give different types of evidence. The hierarchy suggests that quantitative studies, and in particular RCTs, are stronger than qualitative studies. However, this is not always the case; it depends what you are trying to find out – you cannot find everything out using an RCT or even quantitative research. **For example**, if you want to know whether a particular intervention is successful – such as providing day care for children at risk, or using a new type of leg ulcer dressing – you need a study that directly compares one intervention with another. In other words, comparing two types of day care, *or* comparing day care with staying at home, *or* comparing different types of leg ulcer dressings. This would probably be an RCT.

The most common type of study for finding out whether an intervention is successful or not is an RCT or a similar quantitative study; so the hierarchy does 'work' on this occasion. However, RCTs would not be useful if you were aiming to find out about clients' experience of day care or patients' views about the new leg ulcer dressing. A direct comparison of the effectiveness of either day care or dressings will not tell you about what the care or treatment was like for the patient or client. In order to find out about this you will usually need qualitative research. Therefore the 'traditional' hierarchy of evidence is only helpful for assessing strength of evidence in certain situations.

A rough hierarchy of evidence when looking at patient or client experiences is as follows.

Systematic reviews of research

Qualitative research

Anecdotal reports

So, there is no such thing as one hierarchy of evidence that works for all situations. Beware of any literature that describes one hierarchy of evidence as if there is *only* one. Your question should be 'What type of evidence do I need for my question?' It is far better to work out what type of evidence you need for your particular topic and then make up your own 'hierarchy of evidence' for what you are looking for (Aveyard 2010).

Qualitative research

If you are trying to find out about patients' or clients' experiences, such as how they feel about their care, or what it is like to live with a particular condition, then you need to look for qualitative research. This is because qualitative research explores topics through discussion with people involved in the situation, often using interviews or group interviews. Qualitative research is used to explore topics which cannot be measured numerically. **For example**, the question 'What is it like to move to the UK as a political refugee?' is one that would be answered by obtaining in-depth responses from the refugees themselves through in-depth interviews. Qualitative research studies tend to use smaller numbers of participants than quantitative studies.

The aim of all qualitative approaches is to **explore the meaning** *of and develop* **in-depth understanding** *of the research topic as experienced by the participants of the research.*

In-depth interviews are generally used to collect data. Qualitative research is useful when you are looking for in-depth answers to questions that cannot be answered numerically. The aim of most qualitative data analysis is to study the interview scripts or other data obtained for the study and develop an understanding of this data. The data is coded and themes are then generated from the data set. For this reason, large numbers of participants are rarely used (and are not necessarily appropriate) in qualitative research.

Characteristics of qualitative research

- **Depth** rather than breadth is the focus of qualitative research.
- Researchers seek to understand the **whole** of an experience and gain insight into the participants' situation.
- The data collected is not numerical but is collected, often through interview, using the **words and descriptions** given by participants.
- Researchers do not set out looking for specific ideas, hoping to confirm pre-existing beliefs. Instead, they code the data according to ideas arising from within it. This process is often referred to as **inductive**.
- There is no use of statistics in qualitative research; the results are **descriptive and interpretative**.
- **Sample sizes tend to be small**. A small sample is required because in-depth understanding (rather than statistical analysis) is sought from information-rich participants who take part.
- Qualitative studies are not directly generalizable in a statistical sense (see the section on statistics later in this chapter) but their results can be used and interpreted by others. This is sometimes called **transferability**.

Quantitative research

 If you are looking to find out about a treatment or intervention that can be directly measured, or you need to find out if something works well or not, then you need to look for quantitative research.

This is because quantitative research (sometimes called positivist research) uses numerical measurement to explore research questions. **For example**, the question 'Does nicotine replacement therapy help people stop smoking?' can be answered numerically by counting the number of people who stop smoking when using nicotine replacement therapy compared to those who don't. Qualitative research studies tend to involve larger numbers of participants.

Characteristics of quantitative research

- Quantitative studies use methods of data collection that involve **measuring**: size, amount, scales, frequency (e.g. how many?, how much?, how often?).

- They try to be **objective**.
- Data is analysed using **statistical tests** and results are presented using **numbers**.
- The studies tend to be **large** and involve many participants so that the findings can be applied in other contexts. This is called **generalizability**.

Some examples of qualitative and quantitative research

It is important to have a clear idea in your mind about the differences between qualitative and quantitative research. To get you used to thinking about the differences, we have given some examples of topics you may want to find out about. Read each example carefully and decide whether you would be looking for qualitative or quantitative research to address each question. The answers are given below.

Looking at the questions below, decide which approach is best – qualitative or quantitative? Or maybe a mixture of both (multiple methods)?

- *What is it like to be a single mum in an inner city?*
- *What types of illegal drugs are used by people aged between 18 and 21?*
- *Do antibiotics shorten the length of an episode of tonsillitis?*
- *What factors lead to a student's decision to leave university in their first year?*
- *Which universities have the highest attrition rates?*
- *Why do patients/clients prefer 'single sex' wards?*

Answers

What is it like to be a single mum in an inner city?

You would be looking for qualitative research because this information is likely to be obtained through in-depth interviews which explore the experiences of single mums in detail.

What type of illegal drugs are used by people aged between 18 and 21?

You would be looking for quantitative research because this information can be measured numerically, that is, the types of drugs and who they are taken by can be measured – whether it is possible to get an accurate answer to these questions is another question!

Do antibiotics shorten the length of an episode of tonsillitis?

Again, this would be explored using quantitative research as this information can be measured numerically. In this case you can measure the length of an illness and then find out whether the person had taken antibiotics or not.

What factors lead to a student's decision to leave university in their first year?

This is not a question that can be easily considered using exact numerical measurement. This is because the information is not easily quantifiable. The information is likely to be collected using in-depth interviews and therefore using a qualitative approach.

Which universities have the highest attrition rates?

This is a question which is easily answered using quantitative methods – attrition rates are straightforward to measure and can be counted. This contrasts with the question above which necessitates a qualitative approach.

Why do patients/clients prefer 'single sex' wards?

This question requires a qualitative approach to research because the focus is on the reasons for patients'/clients' preferences (this question assumes that we already know about patients'/clients' preferences). Note however that if the question was simply 'Do patients/clients prefer "single-sex" wards?' then a quantitative approach could be used.

As a critical thinker, rather than ignore or avoid complex and challenging methods of research as you progress through your learning, look up words and methods that are new to you in a research textbook or dictionary.

Many topics can be explored using both qualitative *and* quantitative approaches; it depends which aspect of the topic you are considering. Consider these three topics and look at how each topic could be explored using either a qualitative or quantitative approach. We give some suggestions below.

- **Diabetes.**
- **Young carers.**
- **Binge drinking in teenagers.**

Qualitative research questions
What is an adult woman's experience of living with diabetes?
What is it like to be a young carer?
Why has the incidence of binge drinking escalated in recent years?

Quantitative research questions
Which drug is most effective in managing diabetes?
How many young carers are there in the UK?
At what age do people who binge drink start drinking?

Think critically about how, depending on the question being asked, some aspects of a topic are best explored using a quantitative approach and some a qualitative approach.

Examples of research approaches using quantitative and qualitative research

If you are finding these concepts easy to understand then you may like to begin thinking more deeply about the specific type of information you would be looking for if you were searching for information on one of the above topics. This will help you to be more selective about the information you require for your academic writing or your professional practice.

> **For example**, if you were looking for information about whether antibiotics shorten the length of an attack of tonsillitis, then you would be looking for quantitative research, but the exact type of quantitative research would be a study which **compared** the recovery rate of children who had received antibiotics and those who had not.
>
> This type of study is called a **randomized controlled trial** (RCT), mentioned previously and discussed in more detail later on. If, however, you were looking for evidence about the types of drugs used by young people, then you would again need to search for quantitative research but this time you would probably need to find a survey which had addressed drug use by young people.

It is important to note that these concepts can be difficult to understand especially if you are new to thinking about research, and refining these concepts further can be confusing. If this is the case, then re-focus on more simple considerations such as whether the research you require is qualitative or quantitative. However, it is useful to be aware of the different approaches that may be used in qualitative and quantitative research, as outlined below.

Approaches used in qualitative research

There are a wide variety of approaches to qualitative research. You are likely to encounter many different approaches to this type of research when you read the literature. It is useful to be able to recognize these different approaches and to understand why one approach may have been selected for a specific research question. Some are just described in the literature as 'qualitative studies' while others are named according to the particular qualitative approach that is followed. Three popular approaches are outlined below.

- **Grounded theory** is a way of finding out about what happens in a social setting and then making wider generalizations about the way things happen. It is a 'bottom up' approach in which data are collected, analysed and used to make explanations about the way things happen in social life.
- **Phenomenology** is the study of the 'lived experience' – what it is actually like to live with a particular condition or experience. These studies often use in-depth interviews as their means of data collection as they allow participants the opportunity to explore and describe their experiences within an interview setting.
- **Ethnography** is the study of human culture. An ethnographic study focuses on a community (i.e. a specific group of people) in order to gain insight into how its members behave. Observation or participant observation and/ or in-depth interviews may be undertaken to achieve this.

How can you identify a good qualitative study?

You can use the '**six questions to trigger critical thinking**' but you might also find it useful to use a critical appraisal tool that is specifically intended for use with qualitative studies, **for example** the Critical Appraisal Skills Programme (CASP) developed by the Public Health Resource Unit (PHRU) in 2006. This is a qualitative research appraisal tool, and one of many such tools available at www.sph.nhs.uk/what-we-do/public-health-workforce/resources/critical-appraisals-skills-programme.

Remember that well designed qualitative studies produce better data than poorly designed studies. Do not be put off by a small sample size – qualitative studies tend to be small. You would expect to see detail as to how the study was carried out and, if interviews were conducted, how these were transcribed and analysed.

Data analysis in qualitative studies is generally descriptive. The findings or results are often written up as themes which describe the main findings. You do not usually see results presented numerically or as statistics within qualitative studies, and the findings are not directly generalizable to other situations – that is, we cannot make predictions from the results of a small study to apply to the wider population. However, the results of qualitative studies are 'stand alone' in the sense that the reader can transfer the findings of a study to help make sense of other comparable situations.

Approaches used in quantitative research

Quantitative studies may use a wide range of approaches and, as with qualitative studies, it is useful to be able to recognize the types of study and when they are used.

Randomized controlled trials (RCTs)

Quantitative **experimental** methods can be used to measure the **effectiveness of an intervention** (in other words, studies that find out whether a specific intervention really works). The most rigorous form of study is the RCT. This can be used to test the effectiveness of many care or treatment options where it is permissible and ethical to randomly divide the sample group and monitor the outcome. In an RCT, participants are allocated randomly into two or more groups – this is called **randomization**. An intervention is then given to only one of the groups and the outcome in the different groups is compared. You can then look at the differences between the groups at the end of the study and see whether those who received an intervention fared better than those who did not. This is really the only way to tell whether or not an intervention is effective.

Other experimental methods

It is important to bear in mind that it is not always possible to undertake an RCT because you cannot always withhold care or treatment from one group. Other quantitative research methods can also be used for **experimental** research designs which are not RCTs. These are often called 'quasi experiments' because they are not carried out in the form of a true experiment (or RCT). Other studies you may come across are **cohort studies** and **case control studies**. These are studies that try to link the causes of diseases and/or interventions and/or social situations. Cohort studies and case control studies were first used to observe the effects of an exposure (e.g. smoking) on the health of those observed.

Questionnaires and surveys

These are studies in which a sample is taken at *any one point in time* from *a defined group of people* and observed/assessed. These studies tend to be quantitative as it can be difficult to get good descriptive data from a questionnaire. Questionnaires and surveys are useful when you are looking for evidence about the prevalence of a particular activity, or information about a large group of people. Remember that studies based on questionnaires and surveys have many limitations as outlined below and the results of these should be viewed with caution.

How can you identify a good quantitative study?

You can use the '**six questions to trigger critical thinking**' but you might also find it useful to use a critical appraisal tool that is specifically intended for use with quantitative studies. There are different tools suitable for quantitative research available using CASP, available at www.sph.nhs.uk/what-we-do/public-health-workforce/resources/critical-appraisals-skills-programme.

Remember that poorly designed quantitative studies produce weak data. In order to tell if a study has been carried out well, you need to know the method by which the study has been undertaken. In general the study will be more reliable if the sample size is large and the method of study is appropriate to its aims. As with qualitative research, look for a clear description of the method by which the study has been carried out.

Data analysis in quantitative research

Data analysis in quantitative research is usually presented using numbers or statistics. Sometimes it is really hard to understand the statistics and tables in quantitative research but there are a few key things you should be able understand. Researchers themselves sometimes employ statisticians to help them analyse and interpret the results.

When you next look at a quantitative research study, read the discussion where the results are explained and then go back to the actual numbers to see if you can understand them better.

Statistics

There are two types of statistics: descriptive and inferential.

Descriptive statistics describe the data or results in a paper. These statistics should describe clearly the main results. **For example**, how many people answered 'yes' to a particular question, or the most common response to a question. A study by Gill *et al.* (2011) explored whether training traditional birth attendants in Zambia had any effect on neonatal mortality. This was clearly a quantitative study as mortality rates can be counted. The researchers undertook a trial in which Zambian birth attendants were randomly allocated to receive intervention training (which included resuscitation) or to continue with their existing practice. The neonatal mortality rate of the babies delivered by those who practised in the standard way and those who had received training was compared. Data from 3,497 births was recorded and the results were presented statistically:

from 3497 deliveries with reliable information, mortality at day 28 after birth was 45% lower among live born infants delivered by intervention birth attendants

(Gill *et al.* 2011: 373)

Results presented in this way present only a **description** of the results found **in the particular study.** This should be clearly presented as such and you should be able to see easily what the results of the actual study were.

Inferential statistics are used to make predicitions. Once we have a detailed description of an event (the more or the bigger the better; we would not be very confident in the results of a comparison of one trained birth attendant and one untrained attendant) we can use the results of the study in statistical tests to make predictions about the outcome of other similar events. We do this all the time in sport. If you follow a particular sport, you will see that commentators make predictions about who is going to win. These predictions are made on the basis on many observations as to who has won on previous occasions. Now of course we cannot tell if a sportsman will win again but if we have enough prior evidence to go on, we can make a reasonable prediction. This is what statisticians do. They look at what has happened in a particular event (such as in a study situation) and they then make a prediction as to whether we are likely to see this result outside the research setting. The better the data they have to work from, the better the predictions they can make.

In other words, statistics can tell us how likely it would be for the findings from Gill's study to be found in a larger population. From these statistics we can then make generalizations about whether the results of the study are applicable elsewhere. You can see why this is important; if we think that the results of a study are applicable elsewhere then the study is very useful to us indeed.

When predictions are made about what is likely to happen in a bigger population (not the sample used in the study) on the basis of the findings of a study, we call this **making inference** or using inferential statistics. In other words, statisticians try to determine the extent to which the data obtained from a sample is **reflective of the wider population** as a whole. They tell us what might be expected to happen in a wider population.

In simple terms, the bigger the sample, the surer you can be that the sample prevalence is close to the population prevalence. In other words, if the sample size in the research is large it is more likely it can be applied to the whole population. **For example**, if you have a questionnaire survey of 1,000 people from around the country, of which 500 stated a preference for holidaying abroad, inferential statistics can be used to determine whether this result would be likely to be accurate for the whole population. But if the sample size was only 50 it would be less likely that the results would represent national views.

When you read a quantitative research paper, these ideas are expressed either as **confidence intervals** or as **p values.**

Confidence intervals reflect the confidence we can have that the sample is an accurate indication of the true population prevalence. Gill *et al.* (2011) report a risk reduction in the trained birth attendants of 17.9 deaths per 1,000. (This is a descriptive statistic, the result found in their study.) They then report a 95 per cent confidence interval of 4.1–31.8 which means that the prediction is that the risk reduction within the general population of Zambia would be anywhere between 4.1 deaths per 1,000 (very small risk reduction) and 31.8 deaths per 1,000 (a much larger risk reduction).

In addition to confidence intervals, you might find probability expressed as a **p value** or **probability value**. The p value expresses the probability of the results shown in the paper being due to chance. It is important to determine the likelihood that the findings are down to chance or whether they reflect what happened in the research.

The lower the p value, the less likely it is that the occurrence is due to chance. If a p value is less than 0.05 (1:20) we say the occurrence is unlikely to be due to chance.

In their study of birth attendants, Gill *et al.* (2011) did not calculate p values; however if they had, they would tell us how likely it was that the difference between the outcomes in the two groups (those who had the trained birth attendants and those who did not) was due to chance or was really due to the training of the birth attendants. Even if both groups were attended to by a trained birth attendant, you would be likely to see a variety of outcomes in each group due to natural differences between the groups. This could be just a chance variation, as no two groups are ever exactly the same, or it could be due to the intervention. What we want to find out is whether the difference between those cared for by the trained birth attendants and those cared for in the traditional manner can be attributed to the training of the birth attendant or whether it is just a chance finding. The p value can then be calculated to determine whether the differences in outcomes observed is due to chance or not.

To calculate the P value we use the **null hypothesis**. This is a phrase that is used when you state (in order to test it) that there is no relationship between the different elements (or **variables**) under study. This can be calculated using a statistical test, such as the Chi squared test. A p value of 0.05, **for example**, means that there is a (1:20) chance of seeing these results if the null hypothesis were true, and is not generally low enough to rule out chance.

Let's imagine that Gill *et al.* (2011) expressed a p value of p = 0.002. This would mean that there is a 2:1000 chance that the differences were due to chance alone. A p value expressed as p = 0.002 indicates that it is unlikely that the improvement in risk reduction in the women attended to by the trained birth attendant was due to chance.

Here we have provided a brief overview of the commonly held beliefs about and ways of presenting inferential statistics. Some people find these concepts easy to comprehend; others find it more difficult and need to read and re-read the points made several times before they begin to make sense. If this applies to you, then do re-read the section above. You might also find it useful to read other textbooks which describe the use of statistics. For those who find the concepts easy to follow, consider developing your understanding through further reading of books on statistics which are specifically designed for health and social care professionals.

Will you always find up-to-date research and information for your practice?

While there has been a huge increase in the amount of available information, it is still the case that some areas of health and social and social care are under-researched. Research is still a developing area in some fields, and not all areas of health and social care are underpinned by a sound body of knowledge. So you might find yourself in one of two situations – either:

- You are bombarded by a wealth of information that you need to make sense of, or
- You do not find any information that relates to your selected topic.

If you can find a literature review on your topic then you have probably identified the best available evidence. Failing that, the next best thing is to collate the available research evidence on your topic. If there is no research then guidelines or policy may help and if these are not available then professional and expert opinion should be drawn on. Although finding evidence is very important, sometimes there is no specific evidence for what we need and we have to rely on experience and common sense.

The following abstract from Smith and Pell (2003), taken from a Christmas edition of the *British Medical Journal*, and written somewhat in jest (we think!), illustrates this point perfectly (and also demonstrates the process of undertaking a systematic review).

Abstract

Objectives: To determine whether parachutes are effective in preventing major trauma related to gravitational challenge.

Design: Systematic review of randomised controlled trials.

Data sources: Medline, Web of Science, Embase, and the Cochrane Library databases; appropriate internet sites and citation lists.

Study selection: Studies showing the effects of using a parachute during free fall.

Main outcome measure death or major trauma, defined as an injury severity score > 15.

Results: We were unable to identify any randomised controlled trials of parachute intervention.

Conclusions: As with many interventions intended to prevent ill health, the effectiveness of parachutes has not been subjected to rigorous evaluation by using randomised controlled trials. Advocates of evidence based medicine have criticised the adoption of interventions evaluated by using only observational data. We think that everyone might benefit if the most radical protagonists of evidence based medicine organised and participated in a double blind, randomised, placebo controlled, crossover trial of the parachute.

(Smith and Pell 2003)

We acknowledge that this research paper is presented in jest, although it is evidence that the researchers did carry out a real-life systematic review to study this topic. Their point is that you will not always find evidence and this should not stop you carrying out care that is based on common sense or observations that if you jump from an aeroplane without a parachute you are likely to suffer serious injury!

In summary

To adopt a critical approach to accessing the best available evidence you need to think about how you can find high quality, relevant evidence rather than relying only on readily available evidence. To do this you need to search effectively and this is a skill that takes time to learn. You need to be clear about what you need to find out. You also need to develop skill in understanding the different types of research. We suggest you look for literature reviews and systematic reviews in the first instance as these will summarize the available evidence. If there are no reviews, then look for available research that has been done on your topic and collate all that is available. You need to think carefully about the type of research that is most useful to you and consider whether you are looking for qualitative or quantitative approaches. We suggest that you get used to thinking critically about the type of research that is most useful to you. Try to follow what is going on in the research, rather than just relying on a summary or abstract. If there is no research then draw on professional and expert opinion and other sources.

Key points

1 You should understand when you need to dig deeper for more or better quality evidence.
2 You will find the best available evidence through carrying out a thorough and systematic search.
3 Look for literature reviews or systematic reviews in the first instance.
4 If you do not find a review paper, look for research papers.
5 Identify the type of research that will best address your question.
6 Consider what information will be most useful to you if there is no research evidence.
7 Finally, look for professional or expert opinion if there is no current research.

4

How you can demonstrate your critical thinking skills in your written work and presentations

Why is it important to incorporate critical thinking into your writing and verbal presentations? • How can you recognize good critical writing and presentations? • When will you need to incorporate critical thinking into your writing and presentations? • The importance of planning your work • How to demonstrate your critical thinking skills effectively in your writing and presentations • How you can use different styles of language when presenting information verbally or in writing • In summary • Key points

In this chapter we will:

- Discuss why it is important to incorporate critical thinking into your writing and presentations.

- Discuss how you can recognize good critical writing and presentations.
- Identify when you will need to incorporate critical thinking into your writing and presentations.
- Explain how you can plan your written work and presentations effectively.
- Discuss how you can present your critical thinking skills effectively in your writing and presentations.

Why is it important to incorporate critical thinking into your writing and verbal presentations?

In health and social care, it is important to demonstrate that you can convey your ideas in a thoughtful fashion. Showing that you have a critical approach to what you read, see and hear will greatly enhance the quality of your work, whether written or a verbal presentation.

Reflect on why it is important for you to be able to demonstrate your critical thinking and appraisal skills in your writing and verbal presentations.

When you engage in presenting your ideas verbally and in critical writing you are developing your ability to express your own informed opinions and arguments clearly related to your subject. In both your writing and verbal presentations, you need to show that you question and analyse what you read, see or hear, rather than accepting it at face value. You can achieve this by demonstrating that you understand the information you use, rather than just reporting it and saying no more about it. This will give your work greater authority.

In your academic work and your professional role you will need to express your ideas and arguments both in writing and verbally, demonstrating that you are well informed, able to identify relevant information and to appraise the sources of information that you come across.

A much higher level of skill is therefore needed for critical writing and presenting compared to that needed for purely descriptive writing and presenting. This is often reflected in grading criteria, particularly once you move into the later stages of a diploma or degree programme, or onto a masters-level course – you will be awarded higher grades if you clearly demonstrate your skills of critical thinking. In this chapter we will explain how to do that most effectively.

How can you recognize good critical writing and presentations?

Demonstrating skills of critical thinking through your writing or your presentations is a skill that can be learned. You need to do this by showing that you can:

- Select appropriate sources of information.
- Critically appraise the sources.
- Form a clear and logical argument.

Have you ever spotted a speaker or writer who was able to demonstrate their skills of critical thinking clearly? What did you notice about the way they presented their ideas?

According to the University of Leicester (2010), the best critical writing (and we think this also applies to presentations) will contain the following features:

- Clarity of expression.
- A clear and confident refusal to accept others' (e.g. colleagues', authors' or researchers') conclusions without evaluating the arguments and evidence they provide.
- A balanced presentation of reasons why others' conclusions or ideas may be accepted or may need to be treated with caution.
- A clear and logical presentation of the available evidence and arguments leading to a clear conclusion.
- Recognition of the limitations of one's own conclusions.

In addition, Wellington *et al.* (2005: 84) suggest that good critical writing (and again we think this applies to presentations) should include the following features:

- *Healthy scepticism . . . but not cynicism;*
- *Confidence . . . but not 'cockiness' or arrogance;*
- *Judgement which is critical . . . but not dismissive;*
- *Opinions . . . without being opinionated;*
- *Having a voice, without 'sounding off';*
- *Careful evaluation of published work;*
- *Being 'fair': assessing fairly the strengths and weaknesses of other people's ideas and writing . . . without prejudice;*

- *Having your own standpoint and values with respect to an argument, research project or publication . . . without getting up on a soap box;*
- *Making judgements on the basis of considerable thought and all the available evidence . . . as opposed to assertions without reason;*
- *Putting forward recommendations and conclusions, whilst recognising their limitations.*

Later in this chapter, we will provide some tips and strategies for how you can demonstrate these features in your own work.

When will you need to incorporate critical thinking into your writing and presentations?

There are a variety of reasons for which you may need to write information or present it verbally, whether as a student or as a qualified practitioner.

Types of written information

There are a variety of reasons why you might need to prepare written information, **for example**:

- Reports for a variety of purposes.
- Case studies.
- Academic essays or assignments.
- Research reports, **for example** on a particular aspect of care, intervention or treatment.
- Drawing up and justifying recommendations regarding appropriate interventions for the care of a client.
- A dissertation, thesis or research project.
- Policies or guidelines.
- Care plans or care pathways.
- Quality documentation and audits.
- Reflective diaries or journals.

The importance of skilfully crafted, knowledgeable critical writing should not be underestimated – the ability to argue a case in writing can be the key to creative practice and to positive changes in health and social care.

Types of verbal presentation

There are also a variety of reasons why you might need to prepare and deliver a verbal presentation, **for example**:

- Presenting the case study of a patient/client to your colleagues.
- Giving a presentation for an academic assignment.
- Presenting a viva for a dissertation or thesis.
- Giving a verbal presentation for the education of others (such as in a teaching session).
- You may also need to present your skills of critical thinking in less formal situations, such as when debating an issue with colleagues, or reflecting on an incident with others – this will be discussed in Chapter 5.

Getting your ideas across in a presentation is just as important as if they are written down. Don't miss the opportunity to demonstrate your skills of critical thinking in your presentations.

The importance of planning your work

Planning is essential for producing work that clearly demonstrates your skills of critical thinking.

Think about the last time you had to write a professional or academic document or an assignment, whether a written piece of work or a verbal presentation. Use the questions below to help you reflect on how you planned your work.

- Were you clear in your aims and focus for your work?
- How did you carry out research into your topic?
- Did you consult anybody for advice or ideas?
- Did you access any new information?
- How confident were you in putting together your work?
- Were you able to express your ideas clearly and logically?

You may have noted some things similar to the following:

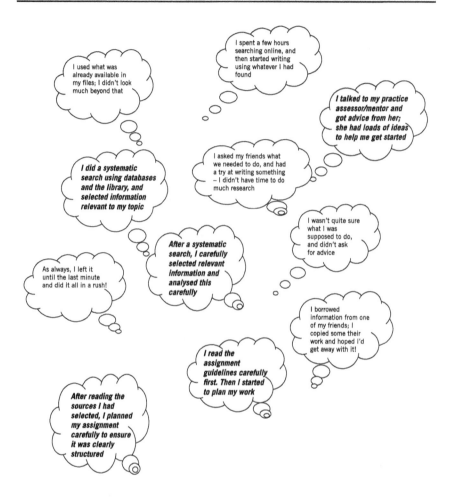

The strategies in bold italics reflect a planned approach. If you adopt an unplanned and haphazard approach to preparing your writing or presentations, you are less likely to think critically about what you write and you may not demonstrate your critical thinking skills effectively within your work. Investing some time in thinking before you write or present your ideas will pay dividends.

You will be more able to adopt a critical approach if you plan your work effectively before you start to write.

Some 'top tips' to help you prepare your work

The following are some strategies that you may find helpful as you prepare your work:

- Make sure you know exactly what it is you need to do. Look at the question and/or guidance you have been given, and read it thoroughly. Underline any key words that help you identify what approach you should take (e.g. *Discuss, Critically analyse, Reflect, Report, Identify, Explore, etc.*). If you are unsure what to do, seek advice.
- If you have been asked to do something by someone on a more informal basis (e.g. writing a report or a set of guidelines, or presenting a brief report), try and get clear instructions and guidance, in writing if possible, regarding exactly what is wanted – this way there is less room for misinterpreting what is expected of you.
- Reflect on what you already know or think about the topic – do you have any previous knowledge, experience or preconceived views that could either inform or influence your approach? This may be particularly important in relation to an ethical or controversial subject. You could draw a spider diagram to map out your ideas, or write out your thoughts, to set out your starting point on the topic – this will help you to explore your existing knowledge, experience and views in relation to it.
- If time and the scope of the project permit, carry out a thorough search for the best available evidence, as discussed in Chapter 3 – don't just use readily available information, as discussed in Chapter 2, unless it is a systematic review.
- Remember to research your topic very carefully and thoroughly – select **relevant** and **high-quality** information that will enable you to offer a **balanced, well-informed** argument within your work.
- Remember to consider new and alternative perspectives on your topic area – don't dismiss a source if it seems to you to be controversial in its perspectives, or if you disagree with it.
- Use the '**six questions to trigger critical thinking**' (see Chapter 1) to help you think critically about the information you have found.

How to demonstrate your critical thinking skills effectively in your writing and presentations

Once you have located the information you need, and thought critically about it, you are ready to start writing or preparing your presentation. There are a variety of strategies that you can use to enhance your work.

Ensure your focus is clear

Ensure that your audience/reader knows what your focus is at the very beginning of your presentation or piece of work. You need to set out your aims and objectives clearly – the words that you use for these will indicate the level of critical thinking in your presentation, for example:

- *Describe, list* and *identify* are all descriptive, and indicate a low level of critical thinking.
- *Analyse, discuss* and *reflect* demand a higher level of critical thinking.
- *Critically analyse* demands an even higher level of critical thinking.

Use simple language

Sometimes the best writing and presentations use very simple language. The author or speaker does not try to impress by using complicated words or expressions. This is a good aim to have in mind. You can achieve this by expressing your ideas simply, clearly and logically. You should also explain any complex ideas or professional jargon and state what any abbreviations mean. In your writing, you can do this by making sure you have full and complete paragraphs that present a point. Each paragraph should focus on one point, and should lead logically on to the next paragraph. Sometimes it helps to put a heading or title for each paragraph. You might remove these before you present your finished writing, but it might help to keep you focused. In your presentations, you need to ensure that you use simple and clear language, and structure your presentation in a logical way, so that your audience can follow your line of reasoning.

Use connecting words

You can help to lead or 'signpost' the reader or your audience through your written work or presentation by making sure your ideas link together clearly (Cottrell 2005, 2008; University of Leicester 2010). As well as setting out how you will structure your work, the use of certain words and phrases can be helpful for this, such as the following:

- **To put your ideas in a logical order:** e.g. 'firstly', 'to begin', 'at the outset', 'I will start by', 'initially', 'secondly', 'next', 'then', 'meanwhile', 'afterwards', 'most importantly', 'lastly', 'finally'.
- **To add to ideas/points you have already made:** e.g. 'additionally', 'equally', 'similarly', 'also', 'moreover', 'likewise', 'furthermore', 'above all'.
- **To explain ideas:** e.g. 'namely', 'such as', 'as already stated', 'for instance', 'for example'.
- **To show cause and effect:** e.g. 'because', 'consequently', 'thus', 'as a result', 'in order that'.

- **To compare or contrast, or introduce an alternative viewpoint:** e.g. 'in contrast', 'on the other hand', 'however', 'despite this', 'nonetheless', 'nevertheless', 'similarly', 'equally', 'conversely', 'likewise', 'also', 'others argue that', 'in fact'.
- **To conclude:** e.g. 'so', 'therefore', 'thus', 'hence', 'we can see', 'finally', 'in conclusion', 'this evidence indicates that', 'because of this', 'my conclusion is', 'to sum up', 'overall'.

Demonstrate your use of the best available sources

Select relevant and high quality research, theory and policy to use in your presentation or writing, and incorporate appraisal of these sources. Remember to search thoroughly as outlined in Chapter 3. When you have a wide range of evidence, compare and contrast different authors' and researchers' perspectives when appropriate, then bring in your own thoughts on these, linking to your own experiences in practice if appropriate.

Make sure the sources you refer to are relevant to your focus and to the argument you are making. You will start this process when you search for information, but it is always worth reconsidering whether the information you use is the most appropriate for your case, as you continue to write. Use the 'six questions to trigger critical thinking' to help you to do this.

Demonstrate your skills of critical appraisal and critical analysis

Give your reader or audience information about the types and quality of evidence you are using. This helps to show them that you understand and have thought carefully about the sources you are using, rather than just using the information that is most readily available. It also demonstrates that you are using the best available evidence to support your academic work. You should avoid just citing a name and a date in your academic work with no further reference to the type of evidence you are referring to; otherwise your reader or listener cannot tell if you are using the best available references. It is important to use the right type(s) of evidence to back up your arguments – **for example**, if you are making a claim about how to manage a particular condition or situation effectively, citing research evidence will give you a much stronger case than if you cite someone's opinion. You then need to let your reader/listener know that the reference you have cited is research rather than opinion.

The following statements give much more information than just putting an author's or researcher's name:

In the opinion of an expert on this topic (Braemar 2006) . . .

As a result of a large scale, high quality systematic review, Jones et al. *(2010) concluded that . . .*

In this small qualitative study, Griffiths (2009) suggests . . .

In a multi-centred, international randomized controlled trial Jacques et al. (2008) found that . . .

In this brief newspaper report from the UK in 2007, Davies (2001) speculated that . . .

When you incorporate critical appraisal of information into your writing, you can also point out any flaws or strengths in the arguments/ideas contained in what you have read, seen or heard, **for example**, regarding the methodology of research studies, or the arguments of people you have spoken to. **For example:**

> *. . . although the study concludes that the treatment is effective, the small sample size and lack of inclusion of older people means it cannot be applied to the general population.*

You will also demonstrate that you are able to think critically by comparing different authors' or researchers' views, and by noting when their arguments support or disagree with each other. You need to analyse how strong their different arguments and conclusions are, linking this to your own topic and to your own arguments. Again, use the '**six questions to trigger critical thinking**' to help you to do this.

Use your own words rather than direct quotes from authors

It is much better to use your own words to describe an author's work than to quote directly from their work. This is because when you cite a quotation you do not demonstrate your understanding, whereas when you put the ideas into your own words you show that you understand what they mean.

In other words, you should *analyse and interpret* (think critically about) what you have read, rather than simply copying down/reading out what other authors have said. This means breaking down their ideas to try and find the full meaning of what they are saying. In contrast, using a lot of quotes in your work will suggest to your reader that you struggle to put what others have said into your own words. It may also suggest that you do not in fact understand what you have read, or that you find it hard to interpret it.

Highlight alternative viewpoints

It is always useful to highlight alternative viewpoints which demonstrate that you have looked at your topic from different perspectives. This will be discussed further in Chapter 6. Where applicable and where possible, you should come to a balanced view about the strength of the arguments you have considered.

The ability to question, and to form an opinion based on a fair review of the evidence, will ensure that both your writing and presentations will benefit from your critical thinking.

Bring your points together (synthesize)

It is important to bring your arguments together, or 'synthesize'. **Synthesis** is the process of building up ideas, evidence and pieces of information and then **connecting them together into a coherent whole**, in order to create new and original ideas and conclusions, including recommendations for new approaches to practice (Atkins and Schutz 2008). This involves stating what you think overall, after you have considered the issue or question as a whole, and weighed up the arguments and evidence you have analysed in detail. It is almost like taking a breath and saying 'AND SO . . .'. You may use similar words to those you use in your final conclusion, but you also need to do this after considering each point or argument.

Summarize and conclude your work effectively

In your final conclusion you need to bring together all the different synthesized points you have made; your conclusion should be clear, concise and based on the evidence you have presented. There should be no new information in a conclusion. Instead, you should be summing up the key points you wish to highlight, and ending with any recommendations for future practice and/or future research. However, your conclusion may be tentative, in which case you will need to indicate this by using qualifying statements, phrases or words such as 'most', 'some', 'generally', 'it is possible that', 'in most cases', 'indicates', 'it would appear that', 'in a few cases' or 'it is unlikely that'. Don't be afraid of stating that there is no clear or convincing evidence for an issue. In fact being tentative may demonstrate greater academic skill than coming to a strong conclusion for which you do not really have sufficient evidence.

Review something you have written (e.g. an essay, assignment or report) or a presentation you have given, to see whether you feel you demonstrated good critical thinking skills. How do you think you could have developed your work further?

How you can use different styles of language when presenting information verbally or in writing

If you want to demonstrate your skills of critical thinking effectively in your writing and verbal presenting, you will need to be able to combine a variety of styles of language, incorporating the best available evidence in order to demonstrate your skills of critical thinking.

The different writing styles we will discuss here are:

- Description.
- Evaluation.
- Explanation.
- Analysis.
- Reflection.

Description

This is where information is given (verbally or in writing) in a factual manner. The **characteristics of and key points about description are:**

- It contains only information and facts. You may use it to set the scene with background information about the patient/client, the issue or problem or the environment.
- Purely descriptive writing or presenting does not contain any explanation, evaluation, analysis or reflection, although it may be the starting point, leading into other styles of writing.
- Description should be concise – providing only useful, important information. **For example**, when critically appraising a piece of research, it is important to *describe the key points of a study* briefly first, before moving on to appraising and evaluating it. When reflecting on an event in practice, it is important to *describe the event clearly and concisely first*, before you go on to evaluate and analyse it in detail.
- In using only description you would be presenting, but not transforming, information; you would be *reporting ideas but not taking them forward in any way* (University of Leicester 2010).

Bringing too much description into your writing or presenting will not give you the opportunity to incorporate evaluation, explanation, analysis or reflection. As a result, you will not have as much opportunity to demonstrate your skills of critical thinking.

Evaluation

Evaluation is about judging and forming opinion, based on a sound argument – this involves the *appraisal* of information or evidence. The **characteristics of and key points about evaluation are:**

- Using evaluation in your writing or presentations, you can demonstrate skills in weighing up the positive and negative aspects of an experience, concept, or argument.
- This style is useful as it allows the writer or presenter to demonstrate skills in evaluating and appraising what they read, see or hear. This is important in all forms of writing and presentations including essays, formal and informal reports, written and verbal reflections and presentations.
- To evaluate well, you also need to *justify* your view, giving a *reason* for your judgement – in other words you need to combine evaluation with **explanation** (see below).
- Evaluation is likely to be combined with analysis and explanation, and it is also an essential part of reflection which is briefly discussed in this chapter and in more depth in Chapter 5.
- When evaluating information, you may want to consider using the '**six questions to trigger critical thinking**'.

Explanation

When using an explanatory style of writing or presenting, you provide justification or reasons for your actions, views and arguments. The **characteristics of and key points about explanation are:**

- You need to give a clear explanation of *why* you believe something, or why you have chosen to act in a certain way. **For example**, when evaluating research you cannot simply say 'the research study was high quality' – you also need to justify your comment by giving further information, and referring to literature on research methodology.
- You should use the best available evidence to justify your views or conclusions.
- Explaining may also involve giving further information about a word, phrase, focus or idea. **For example**, if given a broad topic area to explore, you may wish to explain why you have focused on certain issues.
- You may be asked to 'give a rationale' for your arguments and conclusions within your writing and presentations – this means that you need to give clear reasons and/or evidence to back up what you say.

Analysis

Analysis is about breaking down a concept or an experience into parts. The **characteristics of and key points about analysis are:**

- Through analysis, you can offer a more objective, systematic and in-depth breakdown of an issue.
- Analysis is likely to be combined with description, evaluation and explanation.
- Analysis helps you to answer questions such as 'What is going on here?', 'Why has this happened?' and 'What is this about?'.
- If you use an analytical style of writing or presentation, you can compare different views or perspectives on a topic, issue or experience, and identify the differences between them. **For example**, in your writing or presentations, you may give two or three definitions of a key concept, referencing them. Then, by comparing and contrasting them, you can explain what is similar and what is different about the definitions.
- You can also show how different issues interrelate or influence each other.
- Analysis is a key part of critical appraisal and of reflection.

Reflection

Reflection is about reviewing an experience in order to learn from it. The **characteristics of and key points about reflection are**:

- Using reflection can help you explore a complex issue in greater depth.
- By thinking critically about an issue or event, you may be able to make more sense of it.
- If you write your reflection down you are more likely to follow a structure.
- There are many reflective frameworks available (see Chapter 5). Most reflective frameworks involve description, analysis, evaluation, conclusions and planning, or a variety of prompts to help you think in more depth about an issue.
- In addition to description, analysis and evaluation you will need to explore your feelings and involvement in a situation or event.
- Reflection should involve creative thinking and may result in new understanding of an area or problem you're facing.

Combining these styles – an example

As stated above, in reality, you will **combine** the above styles in your writing and presentations and, having done so, reach conclusions. In the simple extract below from a reflective essay or discussion (it is in the first person, using 'I'), the different styles used are highlighted.

*The appointment was scheduled at 10am (**description**); we had agreed that this would be best as her young daughter would be at nursery then (**explanation**). The aim of the visit was to explore Stephanie's feelings about fostering a child (**description**).*

*Overall, although I was nervous (**feelings – part of reflection**) I felt that the visit was successful (**evaluation**). There are several reasons (**explanation**) why*

I have come to this conclusion. First Stephanie said that she felt able to express her hopes, questions and concerns openly to me (explanation). This demonstrates that we had started to develop a therapeutic relationship, as described by McMahon and Pearson (1998) (analysis). However, we had not yet fully developed a true partnership. Secondly, I felt that this visit partially met (evaluation) the local standards for good practice for home visits that my local authority (MCC 2009) has set out. However, we had not yet set goals as MCC (2009) indicates should be done on a first visit (analysis). Comparing this (analysis) visit to other similar visits that I have conducted in the past, I believe that this was one of the most satisfactory visits that I have ever conducted (evaluation).

Good writing and presentation includes all of the components described above: description, evaluation, explanation and analysis. In addition, if this is a **reflective** essay you may also explore your own and others' feelings if they are related to the event or issue being discussed.

Demonstrating skills of critical thinking in written academic work – an example

Imagine that a student called Michael has been asked to write a short academic report on the following topic:

Discuss the prevalence of smoking in England by pregnant women, and strategies used to reduce this, linking to relevant research, theory, policy and guidelines.

Michael begins to research the topic area, and writes the first draft of his essay, which he shows to his tutor. An extract from this draft, along with his tutor's feedback, is shown below. You may be able to see how the tutor's comments link to the '**six questions to trigger critical thinking**' and to the language styles listed in this chapter. The numbers in the extract refer to the tutor comments below the extract.

Extract 1: from Michael's *first draft* of his assignment

According to Action on Smoking and Health[1] (2010), just over 24 per cent of adults smoke. It is a well known fact[2] that smoking in pregnancy is detrimental to the health of both pregnant women and their unborn children. Experts state[3] that smoking during pregnancy can cause miscarriage, stillbirth and under-developed babies, and can also increase the risk of cot death. According to Booth (2010),[4] children of women who smoke during pregnancy are also far more likely to be ill more often and are also much more likely to end up in hospital during the early stages of their lives.

It is essential, therefore, that all smokers who find themselves to be pregnant should be encouraged to quit smoking. According to Halvorsen (2008) and O'Connell (2009)[5] there are many ways to give up smoking, for example the use of nicotine replacement therapy (NRT) via patches, gum, inhalators, lozenges or nasal sprays.[6] A variety of strategies can be used to deal with cravings, such as chewing gum, having a healthy drink or snack, or using some form of meditation, or focusing on the positive impact that giving up smoking will have on the foetus's health and development.[7]

Recent guidelines[8] state that women should be given a carbon monoxide breath test when they first book into maternity services, and should be asked if they smoke.[9] Women who say that they smoke should be referred to the NHS Stop Smoking Services, and should be given the telephone number of the NHS Pregnancy Smoking Helpline.[10]

There is much research on the effectiveness of different techniques to promote smoking cessation. Recent research suggests[11] that individualized approaches should be used in order to meet different smokers' varying needs (O'Connell 2009).

Tutor's comments

1 What is this organization? Where did you find this information? You are quoting statistics from Scotland, related to the general population – could you 'dig deeper' to find a statistic more relevant to the focus of *pregnant mothers*, in *England*?

2 Who has stated this fact? You need to back up this statement with *evidence* – you need to demonstrate that you have carried out a systematic search for information and evidence related to your specific topic area.

3 Who has said this – which experts? You need to give references when you refer to others' work, and give more detailed information about your sources of evidence – remember the six strategic questions!

4 What type of writing is this? I think this is a newspaper article, and it doesn't appear to be evidence based information. Could you find a better source of information?

5 Who are these authors, and where did you find this information? Is their work of good quality?

6 What exactly do the authors say about these different approaches in relation to pregnant mothers? Expand on this, bringing in more analysis.

7 This is very descriptive. Do authors/researchers have any views about these? What are your own thoughts about these different options?

8 When were these guidelines written? Who has devised them, and how have they come up with these recommendations? You need to give a reference, and explain their context in more detail.

9 What do you think of this approach? Have you had any experience of this strategy? If so, what are your thoughts?

10 Whose recommendation this is – is it your own? You need to be clear.
11 Is this research specifically related to smoking in pregnancy, or is it more general? You need to explain the context of these different pieces of research, and their methodology, analysing them in more depth, linking clearly to the focus of your assignment – *smoking cessation by pregnant women in the UK.*

Having read the above extract, and the tutor's comments, and bearing in mind what you have read so far in this chapter, write down how you think Michael could develop his work, in order to demonstrate his skills of critical thinking more effectively in his writing.

There are a variety of ways that Michael could enhance his work in order to demonstrate his skills of critical thinking more effectively in his writing. Here we will apply the principles of how to write critically and the 'top tips' we mentioned earlier in this chapter to this example.

In order to enhance his work Michael could:

- **Plan his work more effectively before he starts.**
- **Clearly identify the focus of his assignment.** Michael needs to start by analysing the assignment title/guidelines. He needs to note the key words within the title: for this assignment, he needs keep his focus on *pregnant women* who *smoke* within *England*; and on discussing *strategies for promoting cessation* within this specific group of people. By doing this, he will immediately demonstrate his skills of critical thinking by showing that he can keep to this focus throughout his work.
- **Carry out an effective search for the *best available evidence and information* about his topic.** Michael needs to search for *relevant* and *high quality* research, literature, statistics, policy and guidelines linking to his focus. He therefore needs to have skills in *searching effectively* and in *digging deeper* for relevant and high quality information. He may need to contact a librarian for help with this.
- **Critically appraise the sources he finds as he researches the topic.** Michael then needs to *critically appraise* the information that he has identified in his search, *sifting* through all the information sources that he reads, sees and hears, such as research data, information from books, policy documents, and any information that he has been told in the practice setting. He could use the '**six questions to trigger critical thinking**' from Chapter 1 to help him identify the sources of information that are most relevant to his focus, and that provide the highest quality, authoritative evidence related to the topic.
- **Compare and contrast different ideas/perspectives/research findings that he finds in the information he reads.** To enhance his work, Michael

needs to demonstrate his ability to recognize and compare different view-points – **for example**, among authors, research findings and statistics – and to analyse and evaluate these in a balanced way, where appropriate comparing them with his own experiences, ideas and views.

- **Back up statements with evidence.** Michael needs to ensure that any statements he makes in his work are backed up with good quality evidence such as research and high quality information sources which are clearly referenced.
- **Analyse the information he reads in greater depth.** Rather than just *reporting* information, Michael needs to *analyse it in more depth*, giving greater detail about what authors/researchers/reporters say, and discussing it to a greater level.
- **Ensure that his work is clearly and logically argued.** This will make it easier for the reader to understand Michael's ideas and follow his arguments.
- **Give a clear conclusion to sum up what he has learned.** Having considered the information he has read and linked it to his own experiences and observations, Michael needs to write a strong conclusion.

Having taken his tutor's comments into account, Michael then works on a second draft of the assignment. He starts by ensuring that he is clear about what the assignment question is telling him to focus on and finding authoritative, relevant information relevant to this topic. He takes time to write his work carefully in order to try to put his ideas across as clearly and logically as possible, demonstrating his skills of critical thinking.

What elements of effective critical writing that have been discussed in this chapter can you recognize in Michael's second draft of his work?

Extract 2: from Michael's *final draft* of his assignment, demonstrating a higher level of critical thinking

In this assignment I will discuss the prevalence of smoking by pregnant women in England. I will then explore the strategies used to encourage pregnant women to give up smoking.[1] To set the scene, The Information Centre (National Statistics 2006) stated that in 2005, 32 per cent of mothers who had recently given birth in England[2] said that they had smoked in the 12 months before or during pregnancy; 17 per cent of these mothers continued to smoke throughout their pregnancy. Younger mothers are more likely to smoke throughout pregnancy. These statistics indicate a continued need for action against maternal tobacco smoke exposure in order to eliminate harm to both the mother and the foetus that results from this.[3] However, these statistics should be read with a degree of caution, as smoking may be under-reported by pregnant mothers (Shipton *et al.* 2009;[4] National Institute for

Health and Clinical Excellence 2010); reasons for potential underreporting should be considered carefully in order to identify ways to encourage pregnant women to be open about their smoking, so that they can be supported to quit.

There is growing evidence from epidemiological studies that smoking in pregnancy can be detrimental to the health of both pregnant women and their unborn children (National Institute for Health and Clinical Excellence 2010). Whilst the effects of smoking are not the focus of this report,[5] it is clear that those who run health and social services in England should see the promotion of smoking cessation in pregnant mothers, and in women contemplating getting pregnant, as a high priority.

Lumley *et al.* (2009), in a systematic review of 72 randomised controlled trials where smoking cessation during pregnancy was a primary aim of the intervention,[6] concluded that smoking cessation interventions in pregnancy are successful in reducing the proportion of women who continue to smoke in late pregnancy, and reduce the incidence of low birth weight and premature births. They suggest that smoking cessation interventions should be implemented in all maternity care settings, and that attention should also be given to the prevention of relapse. Given the difficulty that many pregnant women have in quitting smoking during pregnancy, Lumley *et al.* (2009) recommend that broader interventions are needed to prevent people from starting to smoke, for example through the prevention of sales of tobacco products to younger people, increases in tobacco taxation, and the introduction of work-based smoking cessation programmes. They also emphasize the need for sensitive and non-discriminatory approaches to the prevention of smoking and promotion of smoking cessation.

It is interesting to note that as a result of a review of 23 papers[7] related to smoking cessation services offered to pregnant women, Baxter *et al.* (2010) suggested that variation occurs in the practice of different professional groups and services, and that as a result pregnant women may receive contradictory advice about quitting smoking from professionals. Their review therefore suggests that there may be a need for greater staff training in this area, and that the use of clearer procedures and protocols for staff to follow might be beneficial.[8]

In June 2010, the National Institute for Health and Clinical Excellence published official guidelines for assisting women to quit smoking during pregnancy and following childbirth. The guidelines are aimed at managers and professionals working in England and Wales in health care services, local authorities, education, and the private, voluntary and community sectors. The guidelines promote a sensitive, client-centred approach, acknowledging that some women may be reluctant to say that they smoke.

In summary,[9] it is clear that there is much effort taking place to reduce the incidence of smoking in pregnant women in England. Health and social care practitioners will benefit from keeping up to date with developments in research and policy in relation to this aspect of their practice, in order to identify successful strategies that may assist pregnant women to quit smoking.

Tutor's comments

1 Good – you have clearly set out your focus at the beginning of your work, and set out your plans for how you will structure your report.
2 Good – this statistic is specific to England, directly relevant to your focus. In a longer piece, you could expand further on this to compare different statistics.
3 Good – you have set the scene for your work with relevant statistics.
4 Well done – you have noted the potential limitations of the statistics you have cited, demonstrating the ability to critically appraise and critically analyse what you read.
5 Good – you are ensuring that you keep your work relevant to the focus of the question you have been set.
6 Again, you are demonstrating that you have identified high quality evidence relevant to the question you have been set, and that you have been able to understand the key conclusions from their research. Well done.
7 This is relevant to your focus, which is good; but do you know where these papers came from? Were the papers all based on smoking cessation services in England?
8 The conclusions you draw from this paper are tentative, which shows that you are able to distinguish between strong evidence and less decisive evidence. Well done.
9 Good – you are summing up your work here.

Michael has now developed his work to demonstrate a more critical approach in his writing – he has ensured that his work is relevant to the question he has been set, and he has linked to relevant and high quality sources of information, demonstrating that he has critically appraised them. As a result, his tutor's feedback is far more positive.

Michael's work could be developed further – this is just a small extract, but if he was able to write a longer piece, he could analyse the issues in even more depth, incorporating more critical analysis of a wider range of statistics, research and literature.

How can you demonstrate your skills of critical thinking in your verbal presentations?

So far in this chapter, we have identified some common principles. We will now look a little more at how you can demonstrate your skills of critical appraisal in your verbal presentations, and how you can prepare for delivering a presentation.

Many people struggle to demonstrate their skills of critical thinking and critical appraisal in their verbal presentations, and lack confidence in their abilities. It can be tempting to focus on **what content to include** in a presentation, rather than on **how the content should be delivered**. But both of these are important things to consider. It is easy to focus on just **presenting** or **describing** the information, rather than on analysing, explaining, evaluating, critically appraising or reflecting on it.

Many of the principles for incorporating critical thinking into your writing are also relevant to verbal presentations, and we have covered these earlier in this chapter. It is worth revisiting them and thinking about how they might relate to presenting your ideas verbally.

Some 'top tips' for preparing and delivering a presentation

Before considering how to incorporate critical appraisal into your work, here are some top tips you should consider when preparing to deliver a verbal presentation. These will help you develop confidence and competence when presenting.

- Check where your presentation will be held and what time it starts – can you access the venue in advance to set up?
- Check whether you have access to, and permission to use, audio-visual aids and other equipment – you may need to book it/bring your own.
- Check that you know how to use any equipment, so that you are not unduly nervous or distracted about using it – if you need help, find someone to show you.
- Rehearse! Ask somebody to listen to you if possible, to give you feedback on the content, pace and delivery of your presentation and to check your timings.
- Time yourself so you know how long it will take; be aware of any time limit you need to keep to, and don't overrun – part of the skill of being critical is being selective in what you say.
- Face the front, so that you can be heard by your audience, and speak clearly and slowly.
- Ensure you have some notes prepared in case you need to give additional information during or after the presentation.
- If you are using audio-visual aids, don't put too much information on each slide, and don't read off each slide word for word – this will make your presentation less interesting and less animated for the audience, and will not give you the opportunity to demonstrate your skills of critical thinking.
- Use a variety of approaches to break up your presentation (e.g. some questions, discussion etc.).
- If possible, you may wish to record your rehearsal and watch the recording yourself – this may help you to see how you need to develop your presentation skills.

Having prepared for your presentation, rehearsed, and taken into account the above tips, how can you ensure that your skills of critical thinking are demonstrated clearly in your presentations? As well as the points made earlier in this chapter, bear the following advice in mind.

- **Be clear about the focus of your presentation**, and keep to this focus throughout – avoid getting 'distracted' and discussing information and ideas that are not relevant to this.
- **Express yourself clearly, using simple terms** – do not assume that your audience will understand complex language and terminology, or abbreviations.
- **Link to relevant research, theory and policy**, demonstrating your skills of critical analysis and appraisal as you do so.
- Be prepared to **invite questions from the audience**, using them as an opportunity to demonstrate your skills of critical appraisal further. Link to relevant theory and research, and link the questions back to your focus.
- **Elaborate** on some of the points in your presentation – this is where you can use your critical thinking skills. **For example**, you can **evaluate** information, **analyse** a definition and **explain** complex terms.
- Ensure that **your argument is logical** and that **your conclusion is clear**, resulting from the process of synthesis.

Checklist for assessing your critical thinking in written work

It is important to apply the same rigour to your own writing and presenting, as you do when analysing source materials. Below is a simple checklist to help you ensure you are demonstrating your skills of critical thinking in your writing and presentations. It can help you to see how you can develop your work further. You can also ask your peers to critically appraise your work using this checklist and give you feedback – you may get fresh ideas about how you can enhance your work.

A checklist for assessing your critical thinking in written work and presentations	Yes	No	Not sure
Have you set out clear aims for your work?			
Have you explained your focus clearly to the reader/listener? Have you kept to this focus throughout your work?			
Have you selected sources of information that are relevant to the focus of your work?			
Have you chosen high quality sources of information, and justified your choice of these in your work?			
Have you demonstrated your skills of critical appraisal of research and other evidence within your work? See the '**six questions to trigger critical thinking**'.			
Have you put together a clear and logical argument, so that it is easy to follow your ideas?			
Have you demonstrated your ability to compare and contrast different authors'/researchers'/policy-makers' perspectives in a balanced way in your work?			
Have you put authors'/researchers' ideas into your own words, to demonstrate your own understanding of their ideas?			
Have you appraised authors'/researchers' findings, ideas and perspectives in a balanced way, even when these contradict your own?			
Have you given references for all the sources of information you have referred to?			
Have you referenced all resources you have referred to in a systematic way in your text/presentation and in your reference list?			
Is your conclusion clear, and based on the evidence you refer to in your work?			
Can you think of any ways that you could develop your work further? If so, note your ideas:			

In summary

In this chapter we have discussed why it is important to incorporate critical thinking into your writing and presentations. We have explained how you can recognize critical thinking in your writing and presentations. We have also explored how you can plan your written work and presentations effectively. Finally, we have discussed how you can present your critical thinking skills effectively in your writing and verbal presentations. We have given some examples of critical writing for you to look at, to help you see how you can develop your writing skills further. We have also provided some top tips and a checklist to help you to plan your writing and your verbal presentations, and to help you demonstrate your ability to be critical in your work.

Key points

1 Incorporating a critical approach in your writing and presentations will demonstrate that you are well informed, and that you are able to identify relevant information and appraise the sources of information that you come across.
2 You will be more able to adopt a critical approach if you plan your work effectively before you start to write or put together your presentation.
3 Remember that planning includes undertaking a systematic search of the literature and being critical of what you find, using our '**six questions to trigger critical thinking**' (see Chapter 1).
4 When citing a reference, try to give some information about the quality of the source and why it backs up the point you are making. Note the quality and type of source, **for example** is it research- or opinion-based?
5 Ensure that your work is logically structured and well argued.
6 Seek feedback on your writing and your presentations from those around you, and critically appraise your own work to help you to develop it further.

5

How you can adopt critical thinking in your professional practice

The professional context of critical thinking • How you can think critically about the influences on your professional practice: routine, relying on your experience and learning from others • How you can identify and use the skills of critical thinking in your professional practice • How you can develop a more in-depth approach to critical thinking in your practice
• How to identify and influence whether your organization (or placement area) has a critical approach to thinking, learning and development
• In summary • Key points

In this chapter we will:

- Discuss the context and complexity of critical thinking in professional practice.
- Explore how you can think critically about routine, relying on your experience and learning from others.
- Discuss how you can identify and use skills for critical thinking within your practice.
- Examine how you can develop a more in-depth approach to critical thinking.
- Enable you to identify whether your workplace/placement has a critical approach to learning and development and discuss how to influence it.

The professional context of critical thinking

As discussed in Chapter 1, critical thinking is an approach as well as an attitude. It is about being curious, investigative, analytical and questioning. These traits and characteristics need to be adopted in your clinical and professional practice as well as in your approach to reading and appraising information and research findings. Therefore, in the health and social care professions, there is little point in being able to understand and critically appraise sources of evidence (see Chapters 2 and 3), or in being skilled at using critical thinking in your writing and presenting (see Chapter 4), if it makes no difference to the management or care of your patients/clients. What is important is that, as a qualified professional or student, you adopt a critical thinking approach in your everyday practice.

We referred to Price and Harrington's (2010: 8) detailed definition of critical thinking in Chapter 1, but it is the latter part of their definition that connects more explicitly with professional practice: They say that critical thinking enables us:

> ... to function as a knowledgeable doer – someone who selects, combines, judges and uses information in order to proceed in a professional manner.

This is particularly pertinent as it asserts that we need to adopt the skills of critical thinking in order to practise professionally. Our professional bodies make a clear connection with this in their standards of professional and ethical conduct.

Dawes *et al.* (2005: 3), in their consensus statement on evidence-based practice, agree that:

> It is a minimum requirement that all practitioners understand the principles of evidence-based practice, implement evidence-based policies, and have a **critical attitude** to their own practice and to evidence.

They go on to say that without such skills and attitudes, professionals will find it a challenge to provide best practice.

What do the professional bodies say?

Access the standards or guidelines from your own professional body to see what they say about the need to be a critical thinker in professional practice.

The Health Professions Council (HPC 2008), the Nursing and Midwifery Council (NMC 2008) and the General Social Care Council (GSCC) (2010) all state in their codes of practice that professionals need to ensure their practice is **safe and effective**. The HPC (2008) adds that if you make informed, reasonable and professional judgements in the best interests of service users, you are likely to meet the standards of your profession. Here is a recognition that the judgement of professionals is an essential part of the care process. This involves critical thinking. The GSCC (2010) adds that social care workers are accountable for the quality of their work and responsible for keeping their knowledge and skills up to date.

The NMC (2010), in its 'essential skills clusters' has identified that in order to offer holistic care and a range of treatment options, a newly-registered nurse should:

- Question.
- Critically appraise evidence.
- Take into account ethical considerations.
- Take into account the individual preferences of the person receiving care.
- Use evidence to support arguments.

These characteristics clearly relate to critical thinking.

The NMC (2008) gives further guidance on this by stating that nurses and midwives should participate in appropriate learning and practice activities to maintain and develop their competence and performance. Consider the following question:

How do you know whether your practice is safe, effective, relevant, appropriate and also acceptable to the patient/client? Jot down your initial thoughts on this.

In this chapter we will encourage you to consider your own and others' attitudes to critical thinking in professional practice. We will start by identifying the skills needed and approaches to critical thinking from the individual's perspective, and then explore organizations' approaches to critical thinking and learning (this could be in a hospital, care home, day centre, office or educational environment). We then move on to broadly consider critical thinking in professional practice. In Chapter 6 we will discuss the wider and more global impact of critical thinking.

You may also want to consider whether there is an emphasis on critical thinking, evidence-based practice and accountability in the current pre-registration curriculum for your profession. You can usually establish this from your professional body website. If you are qualified, you may want to see whether, and if so how, this emphasis has changed over time.

The complexity of professional practice

The real world of professional practice is very different from academic writing and presenting. In your academic work, as an individual, you should be using the best available information you have to make an informed argument. Now enter the world of practice and it is an entirely different picture. In addition to all the information that is available to you, there are many other influences on professional practice which is set in a constantly changing, dynamic environment. All this will have an impact on the way in which you can think critically about the context in which you are working. We will now consider how you can think critically about **routine**, your **own experience** and the influence and **experience of others**.

How you can think critically about the influences on your professional practice: routine, relying on your experience and learning from others

Before you read this section, take some time now to consider whether or not you adopt a critical approach to the influences on your professional practice – for **example**, *do you follow routines, or rely on your own or others' experiences, without question?*

Thinking critically about routine

In our day-to-day working lives (as a student or a professional) it is easy to adopt the practices that have been used by those more experienced than ourselves and to adopt without question the way things have 'always been done'.

Using the table below, **think about some recent working days/practice shifts** *and assess on a scale of 1–5 to what extent you feel you demonstrate a critical attitude/approach to your practice.*

Approaches to practice: 'routine or critical thinking'						
◀——————— Identify where your practice lies ———————▶						
Mark yourself 1–5						
	1	2	3	4	5	
I do as I am told to do and keep to the routine						I often challenge the routine and try to be flexible in how I work to meet the needs of my clients
I do as I have been taught in the past						I am proactive in seeking out new practices
I see my work as a job						I see my work as a profession with responsibilities
I would not feel confident questioning the ideas or practices of others						I am able to confidently question the ideas/practices of others
I would be upset or angry if someone questioned what I did						I welcome challenge of my practice
I only attend mandatory training and development, even when other opportunities for development are available to me						I proactively seek out and take up opportunities to attend a wide range of development activities
I have not read research or new policy in the last 12 months						I have read a variety of research and/or new policy in the last 12 months
I avoid offering more than basic explanations for my decisions						I feel confident explaining the reasons for my decisions
I rarely access a book, journal or professional online resources						I often look up new knowledge in books, journals or professional online resources
I forget about work once I have finished my day/shift						I often reflect on my day/shift
I rarely ask for feedback on my practice						I regularly ask colleagues for feedback on my practice

If in the main you scored yourself 4 or 5 then you are probably **thinking critically** about your practice. If you tended towards scoring yourself 1, 2 or 3 (the left-hand statements) then you may be adopting more routinized, and therefore less critical, approaches to your practice. In either case, you may want to consider how you might further develop a critical approach by reading the 'top tips' later in this chapter.

Facione (2011a: 13) offers a 'critical thinking disposition self-rating form' that can help you identify whether you have a positive or hostile approach to critical thinking based on your actions in the previous few days. This can be accessed at www.insightassessment.com/pdf_files/What&Why2010.pdf. Cottrell (2005) also offers a self-evaluation tool for assessing your knowledge, skills and attitudes to critical thinking.

See if you can recognize which of the quotes below may indicate a routine and unquestioning approach to practice.

'This is how we do it here.'
'We have always done it like this.'
'In my experience . . .'
'I do the same as my colleagues so it must be all right.'
'No one has complained.'
'I regularly look things up on the internet if I am not sure.'
'I heard about it at a conference/seminar.'
'It is in the guidelines/policy/standards.'
'I don't really have a say in how it's done.'
'A student told me this is how they are taught.'
'A practice assessor/mentor told me this is how they do it!'
'I have got a really "difficult" student who asks questions all the time.'
'We can't use the best . . . we don't have the money for it.'

There is no right answer for the each of the quotes above, and we could say for all of them that 'it depends'. If we have considered things critically then our practice should be safe and effective. **For example**, 'doing the same as colleagues' may indeed be best practice, *if you have questioned* what informed their practice. It is fine to 'follow policy and guidelines' if we have *thought critically* about how up to date and relevant they are. However, if you just do as someone told you to do without question then you would *not be thinking critically.* **For example**, imagine the following scenario.

Scenario: John

John (a health or social care professional) loves his job, works with a great team of people and is respected and liked by his patients/clients and colleagues. He works hard, is well liked and responds to requests for help from colleagues. His practice has not changed much in the last three years and he feels very comfortable in his role.

He then decides to go on a course and meets other professionals in similar roles to his own. He discusses his working practices and through sharing ideas and the content of the course, discovers that several interventions or approaches he has been using are out of date. He realizes that these may have been delaying the recovery or support of his patients/clients. It was only through discussion with colleagues and by finding new information that he was able to challenge his approach to his work and become more critical about his practice.

Being comfortable in your work may indicate that you are settled into a routine and adopting a ritualistic approach. This may mean you are not thinking critically.

There are some **good things about routine working**:

- It gives structure to your day.
- You may feel comfortable and in control, knowing what to expect.
- It can improve efficiency of tasks.
- You and your colleagues can work out time frames and know what to expect from each other.
- Where new staff members join a team, it can make it easier for them to 'pick up' what needs to be done, where and how.

Biley and Wright (1997), in an article defending ritual and routine, comment that some routine practices which may not appear to be beneficial may have healing effects, hidden functions or ritualistic symbolism and so should not be dismissed too readily. They give the example of lengthy times for preoperative starving and point out that this may in fact give the patient time to prepare psychologically for surgery. They suggest that we could perhaps create new rituals and rediscover that some older rituals might actually have been beneficial. We often hear the comment, 'don't throw the baby out with the bathwater', and this implies that some good practices may have been discarded without fully considering their sometimes hidden usefulness.

Zisberg *et al.* (2007) undertook an analysis of the concept of 'routine' and found that it can be useful in times of change. Routine can give us structure in times of chaos and it can be comforting to know that there are certain things that are predictable.

There are also some **negative things about routine working**:

- It may prevent you from adopting a critical approach – **for example**, it may stifle the development of new and creative approaches to patient/client problems or issues.
- It may not allow you to meet the individualized needs of your patients/clients.
- Your work may become boring and predictable.
- When something unexpected happens, things can become disorganized and people may not cope.

- There may be less flexibility regarding timings – there may be really busy times and really slack times (e.g. if the routine says that all clients need to have a certain intervention or therapy at a certain time).
- It may encourage you to adopt a ritualistic approach to your practice.

Hek *et al.* (2003) assert that although some ritualistic practices might be beneficial, out of date and unsafe practices should be reviewed so that health and social care practitioners can feel confident that the care they are delivering is the best possible. All unsafe practices should of course be stopped.

In practice we may get stuck into thinking there is only one solution, especially if such an approach has become accepted as the only way to deal with a particular problem or issue. Here is an example of how such routinized practices can be successfully challenged.

A change in routine . . .

A patient/client is confused and aggressive in a busy environment and disturbing others. The usual approach used to deal with this situation is either to call security or sedate the client. A new member of staff who has worked in other settings suggests adopting a more person-centered approach and says they have used distraction as a successful approach in similar situations in the past. She has applied her personal knowledge of an alternative technique to try to meet this patient's/client's interests.

Rather than concluding that the there is only one way to deal with a situation, it is better to be open to, and actively seek, alternatives. This requires critical thinking.

We have pointed out that there are both good and bad aspects to routine approaches. Another factor you need to think critically about is how you use your own and others' experience as a basis for your professional practice.

Thinking critically about relying on experience and using professional judgement

You may be an experienced practitioner or even a final-year student and feel that what you have learned from your past experience enables you to function to a reasonable level in your professional role. However, you are likely to be aware that, while experience is a hugely valuable resource, on its own it is not enough.

While acknowledging the benefits of experience, Thompson (2003) argues that issues will arise if we rely purely on experience to inform our practice. These issues are:

- We can sometimes be unjustifiably confident – we may rely too much on subjective rather than objective measures of patient/client outcomes.
- If we diagnose a patient's/client's problem, then we are likely to make the cues fit the diagnosis and may miss other problems or issues (this is known as *hindsight bias*).
- We may misinterpret the likelihood of a diagnosis, if we base our estimations on specific information about a case without knowing the broader and more general prevalence of the diagnosis (this is known as *base rate neglect*: see Thompson 2003 for more detail).

We argue that safe and effective practice is achieved by using your experience in combination with other evidence, which we discussed in Chapters 2 and 3. Just as you need to be critical of the information you have, you also need to be critical of using your own experience to guide practice. When you think back to the definition of evidence-based practice, as described in Chapter 1, you will remember that using evidence, professional judgement and patient preference contributes to an evidence-based approach.

Facione et al. *(1997: 1) assert that judgement in professional practice 'is a reflective, self corrective purposeful thinking activity' and Downie and Macnaughton (2009: 322) describe judgement as 'as an assertion made with evidence or good reason in a context of uncertainty'.*

In health and social care practice there are many situations of uncertainty and so there are likely to be many opportunities to rely on our professional judgement. In order to emphasize the importance and value of professional experience, DiCenso *et al.* (2004) produced a diagram of evidence-based practice which has four elements: patient/client circumstances; patient/client preferences and actions; research evidence; and resources. At the centre of this is **experience**. Other authors agree with this approach, and there is a growing body of literature discussing the need to value experience, not just 'hard evidence'. McCarthy and Rose (2010) discuss the concept of **values-based care** and explore the dominance of science and evidence-based practice. They express concern that professional expertise is becoming devalued and assert that professional judgement (combining expertise and intuition), based on reflection, is a crucial factor in delivering the best care to service users. Olsen (2000) describes values-based care as a blending of the values of the user and the professional, creating a true partnership.

However, if you are working in your professional role relying only on your experience and not thinking critically about and reflecting on whether or not your practices are 'best practice', then you may be delivering out of date or unsafe practice. We now offer some ideas to help you avoid over-relying on past experience. We will discuss reflection later in this chapter.

Experience is useful but must be examined critically and combined with other evidence and patient/client perspectives.

How can you avoid over-relying on past experience?

Thompson (2003) offers some useful ideas. Some of these include adopting a critical approach:

- Thinking of reasons why your ideas, approaches or knowledge might be wrong – even when your first instinct is to be confident in them.
- Getting feedback from others on your decisions or checking out what you think is correct in a more objective way (e.g. wider reading, discussion with colleagues).
- Ensuring that you look at alternative approaches/outcomes to the one that may appear most obvious to you – this may mean reconsidering if the problem really is what you think it is. **For example**, a patient with uncontrolled pain may have tried many analgesics with limited effect and an alternative approach may be to consider psychological support to help cope with the pain.
- Learning more about the effectiveness of interventions we use rather than relying on our own experience. We should also access more objective information about the occurrence of problems, conditions, etc. for our patient/client groups.

As you can see, relying on experience can be beneficial if we think critically about it and combine it with best available research evidence as well as considering patient/client perspectives too. When you don't have much experience yourself as a student or perhaps as a qualified professional in a new environment, you may often rely on learning from the experience of professional role models. But even when you are working with experienced and respected colleagues or mentors/practice assessors, you need to think critically about *how* you use them as role models.

Thinking critically about learning from others' practice

As a practitioner or a student, you may well trust the guidance or example of others.

Over the years, there has been much research on 'role modelling' and as long ago as 1965 Bandura described how individuals tend to adopt the practices demonstrated by those they hold in high regard. This approach to learning may be useful in some situations such as when learning complex skills or behaviours. Brookfield (1987), Myrick and Yonge (2002), along with Welsh and Swan (2002) all noted that observing a **good** role model can help practitioners become critical thinkers as they are observing and replicating the skills needed for this.

Cruess *et al.* (2008: 721) argue that role modelling is a 'powerful teaching tool' for passing on knowledge, skills and values. They say that by analysing their own performance the role models themselves may learn from the process. So if you are a role model to others, you should think critically about how you may be seen by them, both positively and negatively. By reflecting on this, you may become more self-aware of how you come across to others as a role model.

Think about the people who have previously influenced your professional practice. Did you believe everything they said? Did you accept and copy what they did without question? Or did you think critically about what they said and did?

Although you may learn excellent approaches to your professional practice from others, it is not good practice to accept/emulate others' practice *without question* as their approach may not be the best. In a descriptive review of the literature, Cruess *et al.* (2008) found several examples where medical students and junior doctors reported that they had observed many poor role models. Bluff and Holloway (2008) note similar findings in relation to midwifery students and such issues are likely to apply across the professions. These studies reinforce our argument that you need to be critical of the practice you observe. Therefore, we need to think critically about *this form of evidence* as much as those discussed in previous chapters.

Positive role models possess both professional competence and personal qualities that you may want to adopt. But you should think critically about the validity of what you are role modelling and the credibility of the role models themselves.

Forneris and Peden-McAlpine (2009), in their small case study examining the role of preceptors (those who support new staff), found that the negative influences of power (influence and authority) and culture (the accepted behaviours and beliefs of a group of people) decreased as reflective discussion increased between the learners and the preceptors. This may be because if you reflect on and discuss practice issues openly, then you are not so easily influenced simply by the position/status of those you learn from and you are less likely to accept without question the practices of the environment you are in.

Forneris and Peden-McAlpine concluded that those supporting the development of others need to:

- Be aware of the impact of power (influence or authority) that individuals may have – this may be due to status, role, expertise or popularity.
- Be aware of the impact of anxiety on critical thinking – if we lack confidence, or are worried about negative reactions, we are less likely to question and challenge.
- Invite questions in a reflective and critical way.
- Challenge thinking by sharing perspectives with others.

We have discussed how important it is to have a critical approach to thinking about routine, relying on experience and learning from others – for example, through role modelling.

Can you now think about what aspects of 'learning from others' you might want to think critically about?

'Top tips' for thinking critically when learning from others

If you are seeking advice from colleagues or practice assessors/mentors about an issue in practice, you may want to consider using the '**six questions to trigger critical thinking**' from Chapter 1 and, more specifically consider:

- What is the expertise of the person giving the advice? *How do they keep up to date? Can they give a clear rationale for their advice? What qualifications do they have?*
- Is the adviser trustworthy? *Do they have any reason (e.g. pride, embarrassment, concern about status etc.) to 'bluff' or give you false information or advice? Consider if they readily admit to being wrong or are open to challenge themselves.*
- What are the risks or consequences involved in accepting or rejecting their advice? *Can you check it out from other sources? Are there any policies, guidelines or research evidence to help in the decision-making?*
- How full and detailed is the information/evidence they have provided? *Do you have the full picture?*

We have explored how relying on routine, experience and learning without question from others can lead to a very uncritical approach. If you are adopting routines, ritualistic practice or the advice or experience of role models without question, it is doubtful that you are thinking critically about your professional practice. You may have developed 'a false sense of security' about the reliability of the information you are hearing or seeing. We will now consider how you can think more critically about your professional practice and explore what you can do as an individual to develop a critical approach in your day-to-day practice.

How you can identify and use the skills of critical thinking in your professional practice

You may initially feel overwhelmed by adopting a critical approach to your practice. We recognize this and suggest you start with the following:

- Develop skills of **reflection** so that you can fully consider what aspects of your practice you need to develop and how.
- Seek out evidence and explore the **use of evidence** to inform your practice.

Developing and using skills of reflection

Facione (2011b: 12) describes how 'critical thinking is purposeful, **reflective judgement** that is focused on deciding what to believe or what to do'. Reflection can be done by an individual or among a group of people. Facione asserts that if we are being reflective and balanced in our views, then we are using our critical thinking skills. It is not enough to have critical thinking skills; we need to have the disposition or temperament to become a critical thinker too. Critical thinking and reflection don't just happen, you need to be motivated and determined to make the best judgements you can.

Reflection is a complex, widely defined and interpreted concept but, simply put, it is an approach to reviewing an experience in order to learn from it (Reid 1993).

We would argue that the skills of critical thinking are needed to reflect, and the skills of reflection are needed for critical thinking! Therefore, if we adopt a critical approach to reviewing our experiences then this should enhance our learning and practice. Reflection requires us to demonstrate several of the same skills and qualities needed for critical thinking such as: **self-awareness** and the ability **to evaluate, analyse** and **explore feelings** (Atkins and Murphy 1993). Mann *et al.* (2009: 597) carried out a systematic review of reflection and comment that several definitions of reflection from the earliest to the more recent 'emphasise purposeful critical analysis of experience and knowledge in order to achieve deeper meaning and understanding'. This is because definitions of reflection and of critical thinking generally incorporate active mental processes (considering, reviewing, thinking) that involve some breaking down or analysis of the evidence or experience within a particular context and then reaching a conclusion or outcome.

There are many excellent texts and journal articles on reflection, and for a more in-depth insight it is suggested you read more widely: **for example**, Bulman and Schutz (2008), Jasper (2007) and Mann *et al.* (2009). Reflective writing has been briefly discussed in Chapter 4 and in this chapter we will further discuss the types of reflective writing you may find useful in your practice. Although we are unable to discuss all aspects of reflection in this book, we suggest you consider the following areas to facilitate and incorporate reflection into your everyday professional life. It is a good idea to begin with some self-assessment.

Check out your self-awareness

You may think you have a good understanding of your personal strengths, qualities and skills and perhaps feel you are aware of your limitations or weaknesses, but how do you know if your self-assessment is accurate?

> *To be self-aware is to be conscious of one's character, including beliefs, values, qualities, strengths and limitations . . .*
>
> (Atkins and Schutz 2008: 30)

Part of critical thinking is to consider your own performance critically too. To check out the accuracy of your own self-awareness, you could assess your own skills, knowledge, qualities, strengths and limitations in relation to an issue and then ask others for their perspectives. This then helps 'check out' if your perspective is the same or different from that of others. If many other people see a situation differently or see your qualities and skills very differently to how you see yourself, you may want to question your self-awareness more closely. Most professionals will have an annual appraisal or performance review and this can help to check out if our own self-assessment of our job performance is accurate. Students are often encouraged to self-assess before receiving feedback on a placement and this can achieve the same purpose when compared against feedback. The 'Johari window' is a tool that can be used to explore your self-awareness – see www.businessballs.com/johariwindowmodel.htm.

Invite feedback on your strengths and areas for development from those you work with, perhaps seniors, peers and/or more junior colleagues as they will all offer different perspectives. If you are a student, work with different members of staff and see if they identify similar or different areas of strength and areas that you can develop further.

Use reflective frameworks

There are a variety of reflective frameworks available (e.g. Gibbs 1988; Stephenson 1994; Johns and Freshwater 2005; Driscoll 2007). Most incorporate an element of evaluation and analysis and so, as we have indicated throughout this book, using these approaches will ensure you are being critical in your day-to-day practice. Driscoll's (2007) 'What?' model of structured reflection, shown below, is a tool you can use to enhance your critical thinking skills (see Chapter 4 for ideas on description, analysis, evaluation and explanation).

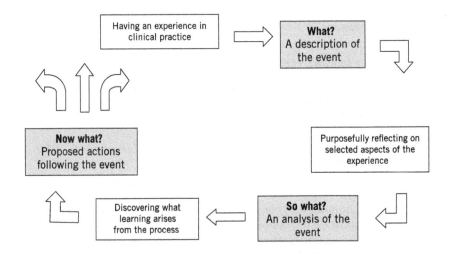

Considering what aspects of your practice you may need to develop

In order to spot what aspects of your professional practice you may need to develop, you can start by purposefully and critically thinking about, or reflecting on, all aspects of your own work, which means adopting a questioning approach to all that you read, see, hear and do in relation to your practice.

- Reflect on your working day using a framework such as the one above, or using one of the approaches discussed below.
- You could try to imagine you were/are new to the job (or as a student/ learner you may be new to a placement): what would your impressions be and would you see anything that you might consider to be unprofessional, unjustified or routine?
- You could use team discussions and observations to find out what areas of practice you and your colleagues approach in an uncertain or inconsistent way.
- Consider and reflect upon what the reasons are for the way you carry out

your practice and then consider how you can move to a more critical and evidence-based approach.

- You could reflect on the management of a patient/client to see how you could improve this.
- Undertake a SWOT analysis (explained below).

In Chapter 1, we introduced the term 'critical analysis' and explained how it involves breaking down a situation or the written word. Although the origin of the SWOT analysis tool is unknown and there are some that criticize its theoretical underpinnings, it is often used as an evaluation and planning tool in business, the professions and education (Helms and Nixon 2010). We have found it to be a useful tool for exploring professional practice. It gives a simple framework for you to consider an issue or an aspect of practice. Often the top row is used to consider personal or internal things and the bottom row for the 'bigger picture' or external influences.

Carry out a SWOT analysis (see below) of a particular aspect of your practice within your workplace. You could look at any of the following: communication with patients/ clients; team working; documentation; patient/client experiences of care; job satisfaction; or management of a particular patient/client intervention or problem.

SWOT analysis tool

Strengths	Weaknesses
Opportunities	Threats

Once you have identified some areas that you want to develop or change, you may want to consider how you can adopt a more reflective approach to your practice in a conscious and proactive way.

Mann *et al.* (2009) reviewed 29 studies on reflection and found there was a lack of research on the outcomes of reflection. However they also found that reflection appears to make the meaning of complex situations clearer and so enables learning from experience. In other words, reflection helps you to be critical.

Keeping a reflective diary or learning journal

This will help you 'work through' issues from your professional working life and by following a reflective framework you will incorporate a questioning approach that will ensure you are being critical. Jasper (2008) and Moon (1999) identify that keeping a diary or learning journal can help us learn from our own experiences and can encourage deeper levels of learning. It can also help us develop skills for critical thinking and a questioning approach. For more detail on this topic see Jasper (2008) who outlines several useful strategies for individual and group learning from diary- or journal-keeping.

Keep a reflective diary for a few days. Use a structured approach and see if it impacts on the way you think about your practice.

You could also identify a 'critical friend' or engage in 'clinical/educational supervision' in order to gain more structured support for your reflection. Sometimes a more formal arrangement exists in the form of clinical or educational supervision and this can be with one other person or within groups, such as in action learning sets. These approaches are now discussed in a little more detail.

Use a 'critical friend'

A critical friend can help you as a professional or a student to make sense of a situation by commenting on and questioning your reflections (Taylor 2006). Appleton (2008) adds that a critical friend should be both challenging and supporting and asks key questions to promote deeper analysis. This requires a relationship of trust, honesty and openness.

Clinical or educational supervision

Supervision or 'action learning' can be achieved by meeting to discuss professional and practice issues in a non-threatening, supportive environment. The development of a trusting relationship is crucial. This can help produce a critical approach to professional practice in the following ways:

- By 'challenging' each other in a supportive way.
- By acting as a sounding board (so you can offer creative ideas and thoughts).
- By asking probing questions.
- By listening to each other's perspectives.
- By offering an expert opinion on a situation.
- By considering alternative options for solving an issue/problem.
- By using the '**six questions to trigger critical thinking**' together.
- By giving time and attention to exploring significant professional issues.
- By acknowledging the emotional impact of challenging professional situations.

Supervision in this context is not necessarily hierarchical – the supervisor is there as a *reflective partner*. You may however want to identify someone to discuss your practice with whose view you respect. If two professionals explore their thinking together it can broaden perspectives and encourage questioning. Kadushin and Harkness (2002) note in relation to social work supervision that the learner should be active in the process of supervision and set the agenda. Bradshaw *et al.* (2007) found that through supervision mental health nurses had greater knowledge of their patients'/clients' conditions, although they recognized that there is a need for more robust research to be carried out to support their initial research.

Action learning sets

McGill and Beaty (2001: 1) explain that 'action learning is a process of learning and reflection that happens with the support of a group or "set" of colleagues working with real problems with the intention of getting things done'. From our experience, it can be useful to reflect and discuss in groups where there is a particular common focus or area of interest. Dunphy *et al.* (2010) describe how when action learning was used as part of a course, participants were able to discuss real problems that concerned them, although they did note some problems regarding participants' commitment to working in action learning sets.

Critical incident analysis or debriefing

The analysis of significant (or 'critical') situations can be valuable in terms of identifying reasons why we act in certain ways or make certain decisions, in order to learn from those situations. The critical incident technique has been around for many years and Flanagan (1954) described how it was used to learn from the success or failures of pilots in flight training schools. It has been widely used as a tool in practice and education in health care and social work to aid critical reflection (Green Lister and Crisp 2007). It can help practitioners to uncover why they may have acted in a certain way and what has influenced their decision-making.

Debriefing is used particularly in stressful or unusual situations in order to learn from them. For example Keene *et al.* (2010) discuss bereavement debriefing where health care professionals use a clear structure to explore specific cases: this involves exploring coping strategies and lessons learned using a series of prompt questions. Pearson and Smith (1986: 158) have a very simple question that can help with debriefing:

'What happened?'

Such a simple question can help a professional or student to discuss an issue, an incident or practice situation in their own way. We have often used a similar simple statement 'Tell me about it' to encourage both students and professionals to reflect fully on an issue. Prompt questions can be used once the reflection starts, such as those outlined in Johns and Freshwater (2005) or as described by Brotherton and Parker (2008):

- What was the context?
- How were you feeling before or after the event or issue?
- What were you thinking?
- How did others see the event or issue?
- What were the consequences?

By adopting such approaches, you are starting to think more critically about your professional practice. All of these reflective approaches are enhanced if you incorporate sound evidence at the analysis stage.

Seek out and explore the use of evidence for your practice

In Chapters 2 and 3 we explored different types of information and distinguished between 'readily available' and 'best available' evidence. If you wish to develop as a critical thinker in practice, you need to be questioning and exploring the evidence that underpins what you do. However, it would be impossible to suddenly be able to give solid evidence-based reasons for everything (big and small) that you do on a daily basis in your practice, so it may be better to start with some small changes to how you think about what you do. Being a critical thinker involves you being proactive in considering where you get your information from but also discussing this information with your colleagues.

Start to think critically about your professional knowledge base: use any of the following ideas to make even a small change in the information you use for practice.

- See if your workplace or placement area has a library or offers online resources that you can access.
- Start practising systematic searching as discussed in Chapter 3, so that you access the broadest range of available information rather than relying on what comes most easily to hand.
- Get training in using professional databases to search for evidence.
- See if there are any national guidelines or systematic reviews on key areas of your professional practice. **For example**: NHS evidence, available to everyone in health and social care (see www.evidence.nhs.uk/default. aspx); NICE (www.nice.org.uk); the Cochrane library of systematic reviews (www2.cochrane.org/reviews); and Bandolier, which has a knowledge library relating to different clinical conditions (www.medicine.ox.ac.uk/ bandolier/knowledge.html).
- Look one thing up every day. Try and use professional and good quality sources of information.

- Visit other similar specialties or areas, and network with colleagues who do similar jobs (at conferences and training sessions or informally). This will enable you to 'check out' what is considered best practice.
- Be open to the fact that *'you may not know what you don't know'*. Exposure to others may ensure you are not missing out on key information or knowledge.
- Set up a journal club. Phillips and Glasziou (2004) discuss what makes journal clubs succeed.
- Ask experts to share their knowledge with your team through teaching sessions or presentations (remember to think critically about what they say!).
- Seek out study days, courses and conferences relevant to your practice and ask for study leave and/or funding to attend.
- Ensure that all who attend any development opportunities feed back to the whole team.

Think out loud

Thinking out loud can help experienced practitioners better articulate their rationale for their practice and guide the process of their thinking. It can also help practice assessors/mentors to assess a student's understanding of a situation, and help experienced practitioners explain things accurately (Forneris and Peden-McAlpine 2009). By attempting to explain to others what we do in our practice, we may spot not only where we are confident and articulate, but also where we may struggle to give a clear rationale for what we do.

Agree as a team to ask each other about approaches to practice

We are all part of a team when working in health and social care. It may be a team where individuals work alongside each other every day. It may be a team that works independently, coming together rarely for planning or meetings. You may be temporarily part of a team such as students on placement for a short period. There are ways in which you can use these teams to share ideas and practices. Sometimes this may involve challenge, but where possible you should try and reduce the need to challenge each other by being proactive in your approach, as discussed next.

How you can reduce the need to challenge the practice of others

If you were working and a colleague or student asked you why you were doing something in a certain way, or why you were approaching a situation in a particular way, your immediate reaction might be defensive. We are often threatened by being challenged, particularly if it is unexpected or at the wrong time or in the wrong place. So it is best to plan your approach to challenging each other's practice.

- Agree a regular time slot such as team meetings, case presentations or handovers when practice decisions and rationale can be discussed.
- Invite students to question you (appropriately) and let them know how and when to do this.
- Encourage any new staff and students to share with you any new ideas, research or information they may know about.
- Consider what the important or big issues are which may have inconsistent or unclear rationale and start investigating what evidence is available relating to those areas.

Try and adopt any of the approaches above next time you are working.

Tactfully challenging the practice of others

If you are taking a critical approach yourself, you are likely to be (inwardly) critical of the practice of others. Sometimes you will feel the need to challenge others about their practice. We would advise you to discuss this within your team *before* confronting others but some general tips are as follows:

- If you see practice that conflicts with evidence you are aware of, discuss what you should do with colleagues/practice educators/students/tutors in advance of taking action.
- Ask others for their perspective on the issue/your observations.
- Consider asking questions rather than making accusations about practice.
- Consider whether the practice is unsafe or inappropriate and your role as an advocate for your patients or clients. Addressing the issue becomes urgent if unsafe practice is observed.
- Before you challenge the practice of others consider whether you have all the evidence you need – might there be things you are unaware of, for example, context, more than one approach or different personal/professional values?
- Access and supply evidence to support your argument or perspective before you challenge others.
- Consider the setting: avoid challenging another professional in public unless the practice is unsafe. Ask to speak to them privately.
- Assess risk – you should not delay if anyone is putting others at risk. *You could refer to your professional body's code or standards.*
- Give the person whose practice concerns you a chance to respond to your viewpoint or question.
- Give them time to respond; people are often more defensive if they are expected to respond immediately.

- Think carefully about the words you use. **For example**: *'Why are you doing it that way?'* sounds rather like an accusation, whereas *'I haven't seen it done like that before, I'd be interested in knowing if there are any reasons for that approach'* sounds more like an enquiry and is therefore less threatening.

Raising and escalating concerns about practice

There may be instances where, depending on the issue, but particularly if there is any concern about patient/client safety or the fitness to practise of a colleague or assessor/mentor, you may need to raise concerns in a more formal way. You should raise your concern first with the person in question and then with your line manager. Your organization or professional body may stipulate who you should go to next. This process is often called 'escalating concerns'. We have discussed accountability earlier in this book and part of being an accountable professional is that we should identify and raise concerns if we see or hear about unsafe practice. In order to avoid the need to 'whistleblow', teams should adopt a proactive approach to avoiding unsafe practice.

The Nursing and Midwifery Council (NMC 2010) has recently produced guidelines for nurses and midwives. Remember that if other people see you practising in an unsafe way then this may apply to you. The General Social Care Council (GSCC 2010: 5) asserts that employers of social workers should 'put in place and implement written policies and procedures to deal with dangerous, discriminatory or exploitative behaviour and practice'. The Health Professions Council (HPC) also has guidance for raising and escalating concerns in the workplace and this is available on their website at www.hpc-uk.org/registrants/raisingconcerns.

How you can develop a more in-depth approach to critical thinking in your practice

Once you have grasped some of these initial ideas, you may want to develop a more in-depth approach to thinking critically in your professional practice; it is therefore useful to further explore some of the key theory and perspectives on critical thinking. We will then adapt and interpret some of this theory for you to use.

Critical people are more than critical thinkers, they 'engage with the world and with themselves as well as with knowledge' (Barnett 1997: 1). This quote gives us a clue about how you may need to move from being passive to being active in your professional life and also how you should consider your own role and potential influence. As a starting point to developing a critical thinking approach to professional practice, remember to use the 'six questions to trigger critical thinking' (see Chapter 1) when you are considering the type of information you have. In addition to this, we have developed the following table – 'Questions for critical thinking in practice' – which we have adapted from the work of Facione (1990), Huckabay (2009) and Paul and Elder (2005), which should help you to think critically about the complexities of professional practice. The questions may help you to consider issues that you come across in practice settings. The second section relates to gathering information and is probably the most important, as in busy professional situations we may be pressured into making decisions before we have gained sufficient information or evidence.

Questions for critical thinking in practice
1 Diagnosing and assessing problems or issues/setting goals or objectives
What is the problem or question and is it clearly stated?
Do you understand the complexity of the issue?
Can you assess the cause of the actual or potential problem?
Are you picking up relevant cues (i.e reading body language or more subtle information)?
Can you invite others to question your practice and share with you if they have seen different approaches to the same issue/problem?
What are your motivations for changing or challenging this aspect of practice?
Do you need to ask further questions of your patients/clients/colleagues to get a fuller picture?
Are you open to the possibility that you may be wrong?
If setting goals, are they relevant and clearly stated?
How will you judge the effectiveness of your decisions and interventions?
2 Gathering information/further assessment
Can you define key ideas/issues?
Have you searched for the best available information, as discussed in Chapter 3, rather than relying on what is readily available?
Could you consider using decision analysis tools to identify your options (e.g. Banning 2008) or ethical reasoning frameworks (e.g. Seedhouse 2009)?
Do you need to categorize, using frameworks or scales (e.g. risk assessment tools)?
Can you identify what is objective and what is subjective about your reasoning?

Do you have enough information on which to form a reasonable opinion?

Do you need to ask yourself and others if there is anything else to consider?

3 Evaluating the evidence

Make sure you understand all the evidence you have.

Consider the 'six questions to trigger critical thinking' as you read all the evidence.

Have you judged the credibility and strength of the arguments presented and are they convincing?

How significant is the information?

Is all the evidence relevant? Reject anything which isn't.

Can you compare or contrast perspectives?

4 Reaching conclusions/implementing

What are the implications and consequences of your findings?

What conclusions might you draw?

Have you got enough information?

Have you considered whether any bias, prejudices or emotions have impacted on your conclusions? (e.g. might you make a decision to act in a certain way based on what it might involve you having to do?)

Are your conclusions relevant to the context in which you are working?

Have you considered the implications of these conclusions for others?

What might you need to consider regarding implementing your findings?

5 Giving rationale for actions/sharing with colleagues

Could you give a clear rationale for your decisions?

Could you explain to your employers, professional body, colleagues and clients why you acted or decided not to act in a situation or set of circumstances?

Have you documented your reasons?

Could you explain why you rejected alternative actions or approaches?

If you are facilitating the learning of others (e.g. colleagues, students or patients/clients), are you presenting the information in a way that they will easily understand?

Examples of critical thinking in practice using the above questions

In order to illustrate how you can incorporate some of these questions into your daily practice in a more practical way, we will now give some examples.

Example 1: thinking critically about what you write

Take the statement 'We work in partnership with our patients/clients'. A team of health visitors may decide to state this in written material they provide to clients, explaining the services they offer. To make this statement without some critical thinking could cause problems if the statement is interpreted differently by different people. In order to avoid any misinterpretation, the team could:

- Decide and agree their reasons for the statement (Q1).
- Access any relevant frameworks or guidance on partnership working (Q2).
- Explore what the team's interpretation of 'partnership' is. This may involve discussion and searching the literature (Q2). They then may want to agree (as a team) (Q3) an acceptable definition such as the one below (or indeed write a new one) to use in their publication. It then becomes much more explicit and so can be applied and interpreted better by the staff (Q4, Q5). Bidmead and Cowley (2005: 203) define partnership as:

  . . . a respectful, negotiated way of working together that enables choice, participation and equity, within an honest, trusting relationship that is based in empathy, support and reciprocity. It is best established within a model of health visiting that recognises partnership as a central tenet. It requires a high level of interpersonal qualities and communication skills in staff who are, themselves, supported through a system of clinical supervision that operates within the same partnership framework.

- Discuss and explore any potential areas of conflict in applying the concept of 'working in partnership with patients/clients' in advance of adopting it in their written material (Q3).
- Clearly discuss and identify what 'working in partnership' will mean in practice and how it will influence actual ways of working with patients/ clients (Q4).

Example 2: thinking critically about what you see

Imagine that you do not know how to handle a particular professional or clinical issue, but you observe a senior and respected colleague dealing with such a situation in a particular way. Before adopting their approach you could:

- Clarify with your colleague the nature of the issue or problem (Q1).
- Discuss with your colleague their reasons for the approach they took (Q2).
- Ask them if there is any evidence and evaluate it (Q2).

- Discuss with other colleagues if there are alternative approaches (Q3).
- Decide what practice to adopt (Q4, Q5).

Example 3: thinking critically about sources of evidence

A student/colleague says they have seen a particular skill carried out differently and rather reluctantly tells you this. You could:

- Invite the student/colleague to discuss different practices they have seen (Q1, Q2).
- Ask if they have any information relating to the approach(es) they have seen previously (Q2).
- Explain your reasons for your own approach to the skill and see if your reasons are similar or different to theirs (Q2, Q5).
- With the student/colleague, search for and appraise the 'best available evidence' related to how to perform the skill (Q2, Q3).
- Proactively discuss with colleagues in order to identify whether there are inconsistencies in the approach and then adopt 'best practice' (Q4, Q5).

From the questions and examples, you can see that a wide range of skills is needed to be a critical thinker. But many of them can be incorporated into your work, requiring little extra time.

By now you may be convinced that critical thinking in practice is key to providing safe and effective evidence-based care. It is not satisfactory to work as a professional without questioning yourself and others.

As the context for professional practice changes and the public increasingly demand excellence, it is even more important that we show we have carefully considered our own decisions and practice. However, there is only so much you can do as an individual. We will now consider how you may be able to identify and influence your organization's approach to critical thinking, learning and development.

How to identify and influence whether your organization (or placement area) has a critical approach to thinking, learning and development

How the environment or organizational culture can influence critical thinking

You may have noticed that in a comfortable social setting when we are with people we know and like, we will freely voice our own opinions and views. A good debate or argument about controversial news items, questionable refereeing decisions, the rights and wrongs of such issues as the use of speed cameras, fox hunting or smoking in public places can generally occur in a civil and yet challenging way. We can agree to differ, but debate becomes problematic if it is stifled by anyone who is not open to listening to others' viewpoints or who does not consider at all that there may be a different approach or perspective.

In professional practice, where we are and who we are with can make a big difference to how confident we feel in expressing our views and so developing our critical thinking. The equality of relationships (things such as power, age, culture and gender) can also impact significantly on how comfortable we feel about contributing to discussions and debates.

In professional practice the leadership, the team we work with and the learning culture are all likely to impact on your ability and willingness to adopt a critical approach to practice.

Drennan (1992: 3) defines culture as 'the way things are done around here'. Whatever our role, as students or qualified health or social care professionals, we all need to be working in an environment that is conducive to our continuing development. In a textbook on practice education, Swann (2002) explores what makes an effective and supportive practice learning environment and states that the atmosphere should encourage the development of critical thinking. He adds that learners (we can all be learners) should feel they can question practice without feeling disloyal or guilty and they should also be able to see staff/ colleagues challenge each other – for example, asking for a practice rationale and debating practice decisions and problems. Both Newton *et al.* (2010) and Brown *et al.* (2010) offer insight into the characteristics of effective learning environments by using a 'clinical learning environment inventory' to ascertain, from 513 and 548 students respectively, what factors influenced their learning. The results demonstrate the importance to students of a supportive environment with a student-centered approach to learning. Newton's study also identified the need for the environment to foster workplace learning and innovation.

Using the prompts below, consider in what ways your workplace/placement area's learning environment or culture may help or hinder critical thinking.

- Is there a written philosophy or mission statement? If so, does it include anything about learning or professional development?
- If another professional or student observed practice in this area, what would be their impression of the beliefs and values relating to student and staff learning?
- Is there an open, supportive and questioning atmosphere?
- Do people readily admit to a lack of knowledge or skill in certain areas?

- Do colleagues teach each other and share their knowledge and skills easily?
- Is time made available for staff development?
- Do colleagues invite, and readily consider, challenge of their practice?
- Is the team organized so that there are opportunities for group problem-solving and decision-making?
- If staff members work in isolation, is there a professional network available so that the latest ideas and research relevant to practice can be accessed?
- Are there opportunities for regular supervision and/or debriefing following critical incidents?
- Is your workplace/placement area audited for its effectiveness as a learning environment?
- Is there flexibility in the order in which things are done rather than a set routine that is rarely challenged or reviewed?
- Are handovers, case conferences or teaching rounds used as opportunities to problem-solve and share ideas?
- Do staff openly reflect on their own practice?
- Do staff readily accept questioning of their practice, rather than getting defensive?
- Do staff have autonomy and flexibility in their working practices?

If your working environment adopts most or all of these approaches then it is likely that critical thinking will flourish. Iles and Sutherland (2004: 65), in a comprehensive booklet on managing change in the NHS, say that:

Learning organisations have strong cultures that promote openness, creativity and experimentation among members. They encourage members to acquire, process and share information, to nurture innovation and provide the freedom to try new things, to risk failure and to learn from mistakes.

They describe the main characteristics of learning organizations as including such things as flat (non-hierarchical) organizational structures which support team working, strong relationships and empowered decision-making. There is a focus on the provision and support of individual learning. Appraisal and reward systems measure long-term performance and promote the gaining and sharing of new skills and knowledge. They add that:

Organisational learning depends heavily on effective leadership. Leaders model the openness, risk taking and reflection necessary for learning and communicate a compelling vision of the Learning Organisation, providing empathy, support and personal advocacy needed to lead others towards it.

This is an important point, in that generally people try to 'fit into' the culture of a workplace or placement and so if the leadership is showing that they are critical thinkers and open and reflective in their approach then other staff are more likely to do the same.

The Social Care Institute for Excellence (SCIE 2004) has excellent resources on learning organizations, which 'encourage members to acquire, process and share information, nurture innovation and provide the freedom to try new things, to risk failure and to learn from mistakes (see www.scie.org.uk/publications/learningorgs/index.asp).

Having thought about your own workplace/placement, how would you now describe the organization's approach to enabling and supporting learning and development for all staff and students?

It is difficult to influence professional practice by being the only 'critical thinker' in the workplace. We now offer some 'top tips' for influencing those you work with in order to change the culture of your workplace into a 'learning organization'.

'Top tips' for influencing your organizational culture to develop a more critical approach to professional practice

- Find out who the influential people are (it may not be the people at the top!).
- With the influential people on your side, talk to your managers and colleagues, or your mentor, about what makes a learning organization and how you can develop a more critical approach to professional practice.
- Find out what areas of practice are inconsistent or frustrating for your colleagues/learners (see previous sections of this chapter).
- Ask students or visitors to your area what practices they have seen performed differently in other areas or with other professionals.
- Involve your colleagues/students in identifying how to adopt a critical approach to practice.
- The move towards becoming a 'learning organization' will not happen overnight and you may need to make small changes, one at a time.

In summary

We have identified that as accountable professionals we all need to demonstrate critical thinking in order to be safe and effective. We have looked at the complexities of professional life and explored the pros and cons of basing your practice on routine, experience and using the experience of others. We have also explained why you need to think critically about all sources of evidence you come across. We have discussed ways of incorporating critical thinking into your professional practice: identifying what aspects of your practice need to change; using reflection; and seeking out evidence for professional practice and discussing this within your team. We then considered how to develop more in-depth approaches to critical thinking and finally we explored how to identify and promote a critical approach in your organization.

Key points

1 Critical thinking is more complex in professional practice than in academic writing or presenting.
2 There are many factors which affect our practice including following routine, relying on experience and the influence of others.
3 Critical thinking within professional practice may be facilitated by using our **questions for critical thinking in practice** and defining the problem or issue, accessing all the information you need, evaluating, considering consequences and giving a clear rationale.
4 It is useful to identify whether your workplace/placement has a critical approach to learning and development and consider how to influence it.

6

Shaping the future: what is the role of critical thinking in the development of health and social care services?

Why is critical thinking important for developing a broader perspective in your personal, professional and academic life? • What are the changes influencing health and social care in the twenty-first century, and how can critical thinking help you respond to these? • How can you think more critically about these changes? • Skills and qualities needed to promote critical thinking in relation to broader perspectives in health and social care • Broadening your horizons in health and social care in your academic work and practice • In summary • Key points

In this chapter we will:

- Explore why critical thinking is important for developing a broader perspective in your personal, professional and academic life.
- Discuss the changes influencing health and social care in the twenty-first century, and explore ways to respond to these as a critical thinker.

- Describe what qualities and skills are needed to think critically from a broader perspective in relation to health and social care.
- Discuss how you can broaden your horizons through networking with professionals and academics in different disciplines, professions and specialist fields.

Why is critical thinking important for developing a broader perspective in your personal, professional and academic life?

As stated in previous chapters, there is no point in being able to demonstrate your skills of critical thinking in the classroom or in your academic work if it ultimately makes no difference to the care you offer to patients and clients.

So far in this book, we have discussed how you can develop your critical thinking skills in relation to your academic work, and in relation to your own practice. We now want to discuss how you can enhance your critical thinking skills further by considering broader perspectives that are relevant to health and social care. A questioning and open minded approach can contribute not only to the improvement of your academic grades and to the development of your own practice, it can also lead to developments in practice at organizational, regional, national and even international levels. It can also influence the development of new theory related to health and social care practice.

Influences on your skills of critical thinking

There may be many factors that have influenced the development of your skills of critical thinking including your upbringing and both the content and design of any education or training that you have attended. Consideration of these factors may assist you now, as you continue to build on and apply the skills for critical thinking to your academic and professional life.

Many writers have argued that in recent years, in further and higher professional education, there has been an emphasis on the development of specific skills, focusing on the development of 'competence' and 'employability' (Bridges 2000; Gallacher and Osborne 2005). Generally, these terms relate to the mastery of 'instrumental' skills and related knowledge, **for example** specific practical skills and procedures required for a particular professional role, or skills related to numeracy or information technology. However, 'higher order' skills such as critical thinking, including the skills required to respond effectively to change, to manage complex situations, to appraise information and to make judgements and choices, are believed to be extremely important within health and social care education, and can sometimes be neglected, both by teachers and students.

Related to this, Sterling (2001) and Bourn *et al.* (2006) argue that students in higher education should be encouraged to consider broader issues, such as ethics, political issues, sustainability and environmental issues, in order to understand their field of study in a wider context. They maintain that taking a wider perspective prepares students to think more broadly, to be more culturally sensitive and to be better able to deal with complex problems in a critical manner.

The contribution of thoughtful and questioning individuals to the process of change and development in health and social care is pivotal to the development of practice and theory. Seifert (2010) suggests that a 'healthy scepticism' will promote better decision-making and in turn will result in positive solutions to issues that professionals may face. Personal traits that are required in order to think critically are, firstly, a critical approach to what one sees, hears and reads, and secondly, a critical approach to one's own practice (Dawes *et al.* 2005).

We would argue that a focus on specific facts, skills and procedures and on a competency-based approach to education leads to a narrowing of students' educational experiences. This is why it can be frustrating to be told as a student 'This is how it is done' without any opportunity for discussion or debate. A broader basis for the education of health and social care professionals is therefore needed.

In professional education there should be an emphasis on developing creative and flexible professionals who are able to think critically and respond effectively to rapid change.

Many other authors have supported this view (e.g. Higgs and Hunt 1999; Simpson and Courtney 2002; Castledine 2010), stating that health and social care professionals should be equipped not merely with information and skills to ensure their competence in relation to practice-based skills, but also with the following skills and qualities:

- Skills for critical thinking.
- The ability to reflect on issues and incidents.
- Flexibility.
- The ability to challenge their own assumptions and ways of thinking.

The Higher Education Academy (2005) adds that health care professionals need to be able to:

- Critically analyse and interpret data.
- Apply creative solutions to problems.
- Take a broader view of situations and of potential courses for action.

At this point in your life, what do you feel have been the key influences – in your day-to-day life, your upbringing and your education – on the development of your skills of critical thinking?

Some important questions to consider are the following:

- Did parents punish you as a child if you got an answer wrong?
- Was asking lots of questions seen as a sign of interest and enthusiasm, or was it discouraged?
- Were you encouraged to be 'seen and not heard'?
- Were you ever humiliated by a teacher/lecturer for getting an answer wrong?
- Were you encouraged to explore and find things out for yourself?

When you consider these questions, you may start to recognize how your previous experiences, both in your personal and professional life, may have influenced your approach and attitude to critical thinking.

What are the changes influencing health and social care in the twenty-first century, and how can critical thinking help you respond to these?

Being a critical thinker has never been so important in the fast changing, flexible and responsive world we are living in. There are many changes taking place at local, national and global levels which are impacting significantly on the planning and delivery of health and social care in the twenty-first century. These are leading to new opportunities for positive change, but also to a variety of challenges. It is worth taking stock of these changes, as they will affect your role as a health and social care professional in the future, as well as your future studies and research.

What changes are you are aware of that are taking place locally, nationally and globally that are impacting on the planning and delivery of health and social care in the twenty-first century?

You may have thought of some or all of the following:

- Advances in information access and communication technology.
- Increasing diversity of populations.
- Limitations in financial and material resources to provide health and social care.
- Inequalities in health and in social well-being.
- Political changes.
- Environmental issues.
- Globalization.

Advances in information access and communication technology

Advances in technology and communication, particularly those related to the development of the internet, have led to new, sophisticated ways to access information easily and to the development of many new forms of communication. These have led to dramatic changes in how knowledge and information can be transferred, and how people can interact.

A wider choice of avenues of communication can be advantageous for many reasons. Firstly, growing networks of communication can enable the rapid dissemination of knowledge including research findings, leading to the potential for more rapid developments in practice and in clinical technology. Secondly, we can communicate in much more flexible ways with others, including professionals and patients/clients, at local and much wider levels using different forms of communication, **for example**:

- Instant messaging.
- Online discussion forums.
- Chat rooms.
- Wikis.
- Twitter.
- E-mail discussion groups.

These can all provide the opportunity for networking among students, practitioners and researchers in order to share knowledge and expertise. However, keeping up to date with rapid developments in communication technology, and knowing how to make the most of these and how to use them can be challenging and you need to think critically about their use.

An ever-expanding variety of forms of information technology has also brought new ways to seek, share and store information, offering us new methods for researching issues that may be encountered in our studies and practice.

This increasing access to a wide range of information from different disciplines offers health and social care professionals the opportunity to broaden and update their knowledge and apply this new knowledge to their practice. Professional knowledge in health and social care is therefore developing constantly. As we discussed in Chapter 1, keeping up to date with all the information available to us, and knowing how to make the most of it, can be overwhelming. As practitioners accountable for their own actions, health and social care professionals may find it challenging to keep abreast of rapid changes in theory, research and practice. As well as this, patients/clients now have access to information about services, conditions and treatments, making many of them more informed and 'expert' in relation to their care, potentially leading them to have higher expectations of the care and treatment they receive. This can therefore lead to challenges for health and social care professionals.

To sum up, rapidly advancing technology offers many opportunities for developments in communication, research and practice, but you will need to think critically about what forms of communication you choose to use, and which sources of information you access.

Increasing diversity of populations

Planning and delivering services to suit the needs of a population, whether at a local level or more broadly, can prove challenging. As a result of globalization, population migration and a variety of social factors, most populations throughout the world have become increasingly diverse in relation to factors such as culture, age and ethnicity.

For example, it is expected that the 2011 census in England and Wales will indicate a rise in ethnic and racial diversity in the UK, with increased numbers of mixed-heritage children, increased numbers of older people from minority backgrounds and concentrations of people from different ethnic and racial backgrounds in particular cities such as Birmingham and London (Williams and Johnson 2010). Such changes pose new challenges in terms of how health and welfare services are designed for different localities.

From a different perspective, according to the United Nations (2009), significant population ageing is taking place in nearly every country worldwide; this again has a major impact on demands for health and social care services as well as on economic growth, consumption and labour markets, and will influence family composition and epidemiology. In the political arena, this may in turn influence voting patterns and political representation. Increasing population diversity will therefore have many potential implications for planning health and social care services in different populations, locally, nationally and globally.

Health and social care professionals have had to respond to – and think critically about – the increasing diversity of populations, ensuring that appropriate services are planned and delivered appropriately, taking the diversity of clients within a local population into account. They therefore need to under-stand different world views and appreciate the complexity of notions of culture and the increasing interconnectedness between different nations and cultures throughout the world (Department of Health 2009; Harrison and Melville 2010; Holland 2010). All the professional regulatory bodies highlight that it is vital to understand and respect different perspectives, values and world views, appreciating the complexities of different cultures and recog-nizing how intercultural issues may be relevant to professional practice – this is likely to become even more important as populations become increasingly diverse.

Limitations in financial and material resources to provide health and social care

Although patterns of public spending vary widely across different countries, health and social care practitioners working in all settings are likely to have finite resources – financial and material – available to them when planning and delivering services. As a result, they may need to make difficult choices regarding how to best meet the needs of the populations they serve (Blakemore and Griggs 2007; Alcock 2008). Spending has to be reviewed on a regular basis; changing budgets and blurring between health and social care services may lead to difficult decisions regarding the funding of services, such as home care and day centres, reduced funding for which will remove support for older people. Cuts of this type may lead to the development of more health and social problems in the long term.

At times health and social care professionals may need to justify their requests for more funding; at other times they may be able to make sugges-tions for more effective ways to use limited resources, financial or otherwise, based on their experiences in practice or on research findings. Critical thinking skills are therefore needed in order to ensure that effective care is provided while using resources efficiently in a way that is responsive to clients' needs.

Inequalities in health and in social well-being

Some aspects of the differences in health status between individuals are biolog-ical in origin. However, disparities in population health and social well-being between social groups, and also between nations, are largely societal in origin. They are influenced by the way societies are organized along social, economic and political lines and reflect the powerful stratifying forces that differentiate life opportunities and social need, both within and between countries. The World Health Organization (WHO) (United Nations Environment Programme/WHO) states that within and between countries there are dramatic inequali-ties in health that are closely linked with degrees of social disadvantage. Similarly, the Department of Health (2010) acknowledges that health inequalities in the UK between rich and poor are widening, and that certain conditions that are increasing, such as childhood obesity, are linked closely to social inequalities. Aiming to promote social justice and reduce health inequalities globally, the Commission on Social Determinants of Health was set up by WHO in 2005 to identify what can be done to promote health and social equity, and to foster a global movement to achieve it. In many countries and regions, strategies have been set up, aiming to reduce inequalities in health and social well-being and working at various levels to influence this (Commission on Social Determinants of Health 2008). The aim is to:

- Reduce ill health, disability and mortality.
- Increase access to effective health care.
- Influence lifestyles and health behaviours.
- Improve people's socioeconomic well-being, such as in relation to employment, housing and education, taking into account factors relating to age, sex, culture/religion, race, disability and geography.

An example of a strategy in place targeting families in poorer areas is the setting up of Sure Start Local Programmes (SSLPs) in England, aiming to enhance the life chances of young children growing up in disadvantaged neighbourhoods. Centres were strategically set up in areas of high deprivation, with an emphasis on community outreach and community development, aiming to provide all parents and carers with advice and support on health, early learning, child care and finances, and to provide them with access to other services including employment advice. There is much work being done to assess the impact of these programmes in different localities, which may impact on whether this service is reduced or cut in the future (Melhuish et al. 2010).

Health and social care professionals, and those who plan health and social care services, may have to respond to inequalities in health and social well-being at local, national and global levels, and may be involved in making difficult decisions about how care is to be rationed. Critical thinking is required to respond to such challenges.

Political changes

Political changes at local, national and global levels will impact on how health and social care services are planned, funded and run. It is therefore important that those working in health and social care have an awareness of how policies are created and reviewed, and that they are able to critically appraise existing policy and proposals for new policy. Health and social care professionals may be involved in the process of formulating policy, either formally or informally. An understanding of current affairs in health and social policy, and an involvement in shaping policy, can therefore be an important aspect of a professional's role.

Environmental issues

There is increasing acknowledgement of the impact of environmental issues, at both local and wider levels, on individuals' and populations' health and social well-being. As long ago as 1987 the United Nations stated that 'All human beings have the fundamental right to an environment adequate for their health and well being'. More recently, the Sustainable Development Commission (2008) carried out a review of evidence suggesting that the outdoor and built environment has a significant impact on individual health. The Department of Health (2010) has recently acknowledged the importance of clean air and water for public health in the UK.

At a global level, the WHO (2011) has recently highlighted the impact of environmental factors on death and disease, stating that environmental hazards are responsible for around a quarter of the total burden of disease worldwide, and that in the developing world one third of death and disease is caused by environmental factors. The WHO also suggests that in developed countries, healthier environments could significantly reduce the incidence of cancers, cardiovascular disease, asthma, lower respiratory infections, musculoskeletal diseases, road traffic injuries, poisoning and drowning. Policymakers at local, national and global levels may be charged with tackling issues related to environmental sustainability and climate change, and with monitoring how these factors may impact on the health and social well-being of populations.

The WHO has set up a variety of regional initiatives worldwide, such as the European Healthy Cities Network in 1997. This consists of cities around the WHO European Region that are committed to health and sustainable development (WHO 2009). More than 90 cities and towns from 30 countries have joined this initiative and are also linked through national, regional, and metropolitan networks. The three key themes are caring and supportive environments, healthy living and healthy urban design. In 2008, leaders of over 50 countries in Africa signed an agreement to secure political commitment to policy, institutional and investment changes needed to reduce environmental threats to health in order to achieve sustainable development (United Nations Environment Programme/WHO 2008).

Health and social care professionals therefore need to be aware of the potential impact of environmental issues on individual and population health, and think critically about how this might be relevant to their practice.

Globalization

The growing speed and intensity of global interactions due to the broadening of social, political and economic activities across political frontiers, regions and continents means that the effects of distant events can be highly significant elsewhere and potentially have enormous global consequences (Held *et al.* 1999). As a result, there is an ever-increasing interdependence between different communities around the world – what happens to one community will have implications for others, at all levels, locally, nationally and globally (Harrison and Melville 2010). **For example**, economic issues in one country will impact on others around the world; and environmental issues in one region will affect those around it, whether locally or more widely. Those planning and delivering health and social care services therefore need to understand the wider context of their work, making connections between local and global events and issues.

How can you think more critically about these changes?

There is clearly a need for health and social care professionals to respond to the above changes, taking into account broader perspectives when planning and delivering care and services.

*A broader view is needed, beyond a focus on the care of individuals and on one's own profession and specialism. This requires a **critical perspective**.*

Below are two frameworks that can help you identify what broader issues may influence health and social care for individuals and communities. The first is adapted from an unpublished MSc dissertation by Woolliams (2007); the second is a model by Dahlgren and Whitehead (1993), who were commissioned by the WHO to identify the social determinants of health, upon which public health policy could be based.

Widening perspectives: factors that might impact on health and social care issues (Woolliams 2007)	
	Example
Social factors	• Inequalities in health and well-being at local and at broader levels • The impact of social background on a person's understanding of social, mental and physical well-being

Economic factors	• The impact of individual wealth on a person's well-being • International and regional variations in wealth and the impact of this on the health and social well-being of populations
Environmental factors	• The impact of local environmental factors on a person's health and social well-being including housing and local environmental issues • The impact of wider environmental factors on a population's well-being, including at the global level • Issues relating to sustainability and climate change
Political factors	• Funding and organization of health and social care facilities – different models, underlying political philosophies – locally, nationally, globally
Cultural factors	• Different cultural perspectives on the meaning of health and social well-being • Different models of health and social care • Different perspectives on how to promote health and social well-being • Cultural diversity
International factors	• Variations in population health and well-being in different countries • Different ways of organizing health and social care services in different countries • Different models of health and social care in different countries

Dahlgren and Whitehead (1993) outlined a thought-provoking 'rainbow model' depicting the **'social determinants of health'** (see below), suggesting that there is a relationship between the individual, their environment, social factors and their health status. They saw **individuals** as being **at the centre** with a set of fixed factors (e.g. genetic make-up, age and sex) which impact on their health that cannot be changed. Perhaps in our professional practice these are the first things we notice when we assess our patients/clients. Surrounding them, however, are 'layers of influence' that affect the health of individuals in populations – these can be modified, and it is perhaps these broader issues that we should think more critically about as we assess and plan the care for our patients/clients and their families.

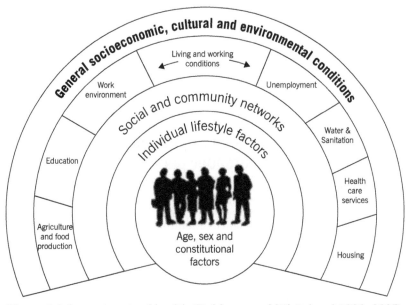

The social determinants of health (Dahlgren and Whitehead 1993, 2007)

Firstly, a person's personal behaviour and their ways of living can either promote or damage their health. **For example**, an individual may choose to smoke tobacco, which is likely to impact negatively on their health. Dahlgren and Whitehead suggest that targeted health promotion aiming to influence individuals' lifestyles and attitudes may be an effective strategy to improve the health and well-being of individuals and communities.

Secondly, Dahlgren and Whitehead suggest that a person's well-being will also be affected by their social support network, such as their family, friends and community networks. They suggest that strengthening community support could be an effective way to improve the health and well-being of individuals and populations.

Thirdly, Dahlgren and Whitehead suggest that structural factors such as housing, access to employment, working conditions, access to services and to essential facilities such as sanitation and clean water, will also influence an individual's health and how they respond to ill health. They therefore argue that improving living and working conditions will have a positive impact on the health and well-being of individuals and communities.

Finally, these authors suggest that broader factors – socioeconomic, cultural and environmental – can also impact on an individual's health. They suggest that attention should be drawn to these factors and to how ill health can be prevented through focusing on them as well as the 'inner layers' of the 'rainbow'.

As these two models clearly illustrate, we need to think more critically about all these issues when assessing and planning health and social care for individuals and communities. You could use these models alongside either the **'six questions to trigger critical thinking'** from Chapter 1 or the **'questions for critical thinking in practice'** from Chapter 5, as prompts to help you to think more broadly about issues you wish to analyse in your studies or in relation to your practice.

Skills and qualities needed to promote critical thinking in relation to broader perspectives in health and social care

As a result of the changes and challenges outlined above, professionals will be expected to have skills and qualities to enable them to work flexibly, as reflective and adaptable team players, able to deal with the increasingly complex issues that may be encountered in health and social care practice. This requires skills of critical thinking.

Facione (2011a) suggests that the approaches which characterize critical thinking include **inquisitiveness** in relation to a wide range of issues, **flexibility** when considering alternatives and opinions, and **open-mindedness** regarding divergent world views. Barnett (2000, 2004) suggests that professionals working in the 'supercomplex world' of the twenty-first century must be equipped with skills to **think broadly** about the issues they face, and to think flexibly in order to solve problems. He suggests that they need to be critical thinkers in order to contribute positively to an unpredictable and ever-changing world.

In order to improve your understanding of diversity of populations you could seek out and take up any opportunity to learn with, from and about other professionals and service users in a variety of communities, cultures and countries.

In addition to the qualities and skills required for critical thinking discussed in previous chapters, there are other qualities and skills needed to incorporate broader issues which will help you to work positively in a rapidly changing and unpredictable health and social care environment. These are as follows:

- **Flexibility**: health and social care professionals need to be reflective and adaptable team players, able to deal with the complex issues they may encounter in their practice. You need to be flexible in your thinking, open minded, able to question your own values and assumptions and able to question what you read, see and hear.
- **Creativity**: this will assist the development of new approaches to your practice, studies and research. A creative approach is needed to your own practice in order to tackle issues you may face.

- **Sound coping strategies**: these are required to assist you to cope positively with complexity, uncertainty and unpredictability (Barnett 2000, 2004).
- **Responsiveness**: this will enable you to respond appropriately to rapid changes and developments in health and social care practice.

Expanding on these, the following skills and qualities will be invaluable if you wish to develop your skills of critical thinking within your practice and within your studies:

- **A willingness to question the breadth of your own knowledge about health and social care**: it is important to recognize that you may have a narrow viewpoint, if you have no knowledge or experience of other cultures. **For example**, you may have beliefs about bereavement that are related to your own culture, or you may select research that was carried out in a culture similar to your own rather than looking for broader perspectives on the topic.
- **A willingness to engage with students and professionals from overseas who may be working with you**: there are likely to be many differences between your own and their practices. Promote positive debate about why these differences exist, and encourage an atmosphere where people can learn 'with, from and about' each other, sharing good practice.
- **A willingness to reflect upon and think critically about how your beliefs and values influence your professional decision-making**: acknowledge that your beliefs will be influenced by many factors including your culture, gender, age, and social and economic circumstances; be prepared to question and challenge them.
- **An openness to new ideas and perspectives from a diverse range of people**: be willing to actively listen to different viewpoints and theories and to consider their merits, even when they are different from your own. **For example**, when researching a topic, you could consider pieces of research performed in a variety of cultures, to compare these with what you find in your own culture.
- **The ability and willingness to work effectively** in environments that are international and intercultural in nature – developing skills to work effectively with people from different cultures and nationalities and care sensitively for people from different cultures and nationalities.
- **The ability to interpret local problems within a broad, international and intercultural context**, taking into account different perspectives in relation to issues and problems.
- **A broader questioning approach, including:**

  Questioning what you read, see or hear, taking into account the cultural influences, the setting and/or other potential background influences.
  The ability and willingness to recognize and to question your own and others' potential agendas and biases.

Broadening your horizons in health and social care in your academic work and practice

Thinking critically about health and social care issues from a wider viewpoint can help you to gain new perspectives and develop your own and others' practice. It could also lead to higher grades in your academic work.

Linking to broader perspectives in your academic work

Depending on the focus of your studies, ways to link to broader perspectives in your academic work may include:

- Considering the issues raised earlier in this chapter within your academic work:

    Advances in information access and communication technology.
    Increasing diversity of populations.
    Limitations in financial and material resources to provide health and social care.
    Inequalities in health and social well-being.
    Political changes.
    Environmental issues.
    Globalization.

- Researching for information from different disciplines and specialist areas that are relevant to your field of practice or your area of academic focus, in order to identify different factors that can impact on health and social care issues – see the two frameworks above by Woolliams (2007) and Dahlgren and Whitehead (1993).
- Researching for information/research from different cultures and backgrounds, including from different countries that you might not normally access, to take into account wider perspectives on your topic.
- Networking with people such as practitioners, specialists, professionals and academics working in your own and other fields, specialities and disciplines, or who are working in different settings, whose expertise may contribute to your area of interest – see later in this chapter for more information on this.
- Accessing a broader range of literature and research relevant to your topic, as appropriate, to take into account wider perspectives.

Bearing in mind the above suggestions, consider what approach you might use to research the following question:
What strategies can be used to prevent depression in older people within the UK?

Your initial thoughts may have included the following:

- Accessing statistics on the prevalence of depression in older people within the UK – **for example**, National Statistics website; searching for information in journals/textbooks.
- Carrying out a systematic search for textbooks/journal articles on the causes of depression in older people, using the strategies outlined in Chapter 3.
- Carrying out a systematic search for textbooks/journal articles on strategies for the prevention of depression in older people in the UK, including relevant policy and guidelines, using the strategies outlined in Chapter 3.
- Carrying out a search for relevant websites which may provide high quality information on the topic, such as those belonging to Age UK, MIND, the Social Care Institute for Excellence (SCIE) and the Department of Health.

Did you think of any other strategies for searching for information, or any other potential sources of information on this topic? If so, what were they?

Now think more critically about how you could broaden your search to gain a better perspective on the topic. You may like to use the two frameworks by Woolliams (2007) and Dahlgren and Whitehead (1993) to help you think about this.

There are many sources of information that you could refer to in relation to the subject of the prevention of depression in older people in the UK. Alongside the ideas listed above, you could take a broader approach to your search – you may have thought of some ideas already. Some questions that might be useful to ask in order to gain a broader perspective are:

- How does the prevalence of depression in older people in the UK compare with that in other countries globally?
- How does the prevalence of depression in older people vary between different cultural and social groups within the UK? Why might this variation exist?
- Do any cultures have a significantly higher or lower rate of depression in older people than others and, if so, why might that be?
- Are there any strategies that are used successfully in other cultures and countries for preventing depression and promoting well-being in older people? Could these be applied successfully, or adapted, within the UK?
- Why does the prevalence of depression vary between different countries, and what factors may contribute to these variations?
- What policies and guidelines does the current UK government promote? Has this changed or is it likely to change with a change in government?
- Do any other countries have active programmes for preventing depression in older people? If so, what do they consist of, and how effective are they? Could they be applied successfully, or adapted, within the UK?

- What factors beyond your own specialist area of knowledge might be important to consider – medical factors, social factors, economic factors, environmental factors, political factors? How could you search for information on these?

You will, of course, need to critically appraise all the statistics and sources that you read – for example, statistics on depression might not be collected and monitored in the same way in different countries, so it's important to analyse them very carefully. Nevertheless, you may find enlightening information that could help you to view the topic in a new way. This broader approach could widen your perspectives, leading to new ideas that you could apply to your own and others' practice, your academic work and future research.

Taking a broader perspective will involve thinking about searching for information from a broader range of sources. However, you need to ensure that that you keep focused on your topic or question, as highlighted in Chapter 4.

Having read the above section, now consider the wider range of strategies you could use to research one of the following questions:

What are the causes of childhood obesity?

   or

What might be effective strategies for promoting smoking cessation in young adults?

You should have identified that you can really expand the breadth of information you use in order to gain a broader perspective on the topics you address. We will now offer another way you can widen your horizons – by networking.

Networking

As well as asking broader questions about your topic, you can also widen your knowledge and perspectives relating to a topic by making links with health care practitioners, researchers and service users based in different disciplines, professions, specialities, cultures and countries. These people may be able and willing to share their ideas and perspectives with you in order to shed more light on the issue you are investigating.

You will find many opportunities to communicate with people in order to share ideas and perspectives on topics related to health and social care, on a formal or an informal basis, as discussed earlier in this chapter. Thanks to the internet, it is now easier than ever to contact people anywhere in the world to seek their expert knowledge and perspectives. Even if you are unable to meet face to face with people easily, for example by attending conferences and meetings, you can still use other means such as e-mail groups, wikis, or joining an online discussion forum.

Within your own discipline, speciality or interest area you may have opportunities to join specific networks. **For example**, see:

- www.rcn.org.uk/nursing/internationaldepartment/international_partners/ icn_nursing_networks for details of some international nursing interest networks.
- www.socialworknetwork.com/home.php for details of an international social work network.
- http://greenerhealthcare.org for an example of an interdisciplinary interest network related to sustainability and healthcare.

Many professional bodies have interest groups which you can join, and these can provide the starting point for discussions and useful exchange of information and ideas. You may also wish to make more permanent links with other academics and professionals, for example establishing exchange schemes with people working in different health care systems and different disciplines, so that you can learn with, from and about each other's areas of expertise, sharing good practice.

What disciplines and subject areas could help you to broaden your perspectives in relation to your areas of interest/expertise in health and social care?

You may have thought of some or all of the following: philosophy, ethics, psychology, sociology, life sciences, economics, politics, geography, environmental sciences, forensic medicine, child protection, and so on. You will be able to think of others. Sometimes you may, therefore, need to widen your search strategy to look for relevant information from these disciplines and subject areas; you may also need to approach experts in these fields.

The benefits of networking: a case study

John is an experienced nurse specialising in dermatology (skin care). He has a particular interest in the prevention of skin cancers related to sun exposure. He has had the opportunity to develop his knowledge and skills in a variety of ways:

- He has joined a dermatology interest group in his local area, linking with other professionals with an interest in this topic. They hold regular meetings where they share their knowledge and experiences, and have an internet discussion forum through which they can communicate ideas and information.

- He is a member of a national dermatology forum open to practitioners, academics and researchers interested in this topic. They hold regular meetings and an annual national conference where they can share their knowledge, ideas and experiences.

- He is able to contact professionals and academics working in the field of dermatology throughout the world on a day-to-day basis through a variety of means, including emails, online discussion forums and by phone.

- He is also a member of an international dermatology research forum, which has a website which is updated regularly with the latest developments in research in his specialist field. Every other year, John goes to an international conference organized by this forum, where he can network with professionals from all over the world.

- John can access information via a variety of journals – national and international – to update his knowledge.

- He has a link with a research centre based in a hospital in Australia which specializes in prevention and treatment of skin cancers. John has visited the centre three times over the past 10 years, to learn from their good practice and to share his knowledge and experience.

- He also has a link with a hospital in Africa where he has set up an exchange system between their team and his own – they share ideas for how to prevent and treat skin cancers, and benefit from each other's knowledge, experience and ideas.

- John has a developing interest in the impact of genetic factors on the incidence of skin cancer globally, and he is involved in research on this topic with colleagues in the UK, Africa and Australia. The team have fed back their initial findings to the various forums and interest groups they are involved with locally, nationally and globally. They have written a variety of papers on the prevention of skin cancer aimed at a global audience, which have led to positive changes in the prevention of skin cancer at many levels, and new approaches to researching the issues related to this topic.

John's example illustrates how an individual health or social care practitioner can incorporate broader, global perspectives within their practice, potentially linking these to their studies and research. This can potentially lead to changes in practice and theory at a variety of levels and requires a creative and questioning approach to practice and research, and openness to alternative ideas and perspectives.

The impact of critical thinking on the development of practice

To sum up the ideas within this chapter, we will conclude with a very short and simple case study which illustrates the potential benefits of critical thinking in health and social care.

Case study

A motivated interprofessional team of health and social care professionals were involved in running a large nursing home for the long-term care of older people who have dementia. A number of staff felt increasingly concerned by the number of clients who appeared to be bored and restless during the daytime. Client and carer surveys suggested a low level of satisfaction with care in relation to the mental stimulation of clients in the home.

The team decided to explore how they could improve the care offered. Their lead manager was fully supportive of their plans, and encouraged them to take some time to work on this project, as well as offering a small amount of financial support.

The approach the team decided to take was as follows:

- Firstly, they met together, along with client and carer representatives, and with an expert in dementia care who was based at their local university. They shared their initial concerns, and discussed their ideas for how they could enhance the care on offer. Each person present discussed how they felt they could contribute to the project.
- Two members of the team offered to carry out a thorough search for research, articles and reports which highlighted recommendations for good practice. Through this they identified a variety of sources of information, which they critically appraised very carefully, in order to decide which aspects they felt were relevant to their setting. They put together a summary of the key findings of their review to present to the team.
- Some other members of the team joined an international online discussion forum for professionals caring for people with dementia. They posted a request for suggestions for improving their practice. A lively debate ensued, and as a result they engaged in live discussions with professionals working in a variety of countries including the USA, Bolivia, India and Sweden. They received some constructive suggestions from all of these people, who suggested many ideas for how they could enhance client care – **for example**:

Involving clients in day-to-day activities around the home.
Staff, clients and carers sharing mealtimes, to promote more social interaction.

Using new approaches for assessing clients' interests and past histories in more depth.

Using simple ways to engage clients such as the use of music, talking books, etc; the staff were given useful information about how to access good resources.

Using a variety of simple strategies to communicate with clients more effectively.

Suggestions were made for how to encourage the local community to become more engaged with people living in the home.

Suggestions were made for how to decorate and lay out the home in order to enhance clients' sense of freedom, while maximizing their safety.

A year after the first meeting, having introduced these ideas and others, care in the home had improved so significantly that it had become well known as a model for good practice in the local area. Staff from other homes in the region visited to learn from their expertise. One member of the team suggested that they should write an account of the changes they had made, linking to relevant literature, and making recommendations for other professionals contemplating similar changes. The publication of this article in a social care journal led to further developments: staff members working in the home were invited to assist in a Department of Health working party aiming to formulate new standards for dementia care throughout the UK.

One of the people they had been in contact with who was based in Sweden asked to visit their home, and an exchange was then arranged. As a result, one of the team had the opportunity to visit some care homes in Sweden. She was able to compare their approaches and share ideas for good practice. While in Sweden, she also gave a presentation at a conference for health and social care professionals, to disseminate good practice, and at the conference she had the opportunity to attend other presentations and learn from dementia care specialists based in different parts of Europe.

Over the years following this, the team continued to develop their practice. They were keen to continue to improve their care, and did not 'rest on their laurels'. One member of the team left to set up a consultancy business, with the aim of helping similar homes to enhance their care. As new members of staff joined the home, they fed in their ideas for how to improve and develop care further. The manager continued to foster an open atmosphere where staff members were encouraged to develop their knowledge and to share their ideas for good practice, and also to challenge each other's practice in a positive and constructive manner.

This case study highlights the value of working with others who are prepared to challenge their own and others' practice, and illustrates the potential positive effects of thinking critically and seeking ideas from a broader perspective when analysing one's practice. It also shows that academic research feeds into the process of changing practice. It can be extremely fruitful to look further afield beyond one's usual sources of support and information in order to gain new perspectives on an issue or problem.

'Top tips' for broadening your perspectives in relation to your practice and your academic work

- **Look beyond the reading list**: don't restrict your reading to what is in your reading list! Read more broadly in relation to your topic and, where appropriate, look for information and research from other disciplines, other specialities, other countries and other professions.
- **Ask broader questions of what you read, see and hear**: use the **'six questions to trigger critical thinking'** from Chapter 1 and the **'questions for critical thinking in practice'** from Chapter 5 as a basis to help you consider the following questions:

Are there any alternative perspectives/viewpoints in relation to the topic/issue you are focusing on?

What have different authors/researchers/practitioners/theorists said – within your own profession/setting/speciality and in other professions/settings/specialities?

What are your own thoughts and ideas, having read different perspectives in research and literature?

Do any ethical issues need to be considered? Would the same ethical issues apply elsewhere (e.g. in other countries or settings)?

What can you learn from *approaches used* in other countries and cultures?

What can you learn from *research carried out* in other countries and cultures?

- **Where appropriate, look at broader perspectives related to health and social care**: social, economic, political, and/or cultural.
- **Look at other work from other disciplines/specialities** to see what they have to say about the issues you are researching.
- **Become more self-aware**: try to become more aware of your own values, attitudes, beliefs and biases, and think about how these may impact on your thinking and your practice.
- **Make links with other practice areas/specialities**: locally, regionally, nationally, globally – share ideas, learn 'with, from and about' others' approach to practice issues including models of health and social care.

- **Discuss issues with peers and colleagues, at local level and more widely**: this will help you to challenge the taken for granted assumptions, beliefs and values that you hold, and to share ideas for developing theory and practice.
- **Consider whether there may be alternative ways of viewing/approaching the issue or problem you are looking at**: consider your own thoughts, your colleagues' and peers' perspectives, and those of authors and researchers.

The importance of people exchanging ideas and valuing alternative perspectives to their own cannot be underestimated, and we believe that this is the key to development of practice and the promotion of positive changes in health and social care. Professionals should be equipped to be flexible, creative and innovative thinkers in order to solve problems through questioning. Critical thinkers are more likely to engage in productive and positive activity due to their continual questioning of their knowledge, assumptions and perspectives. Critical thinking enables professionals to challenge their own and others' beliefs and habits, and not take things for granted. A critical thinker will look to broader perspectives to help them develop their knowledge, practice and perspectives. This curiosity and open-mindedness will lead to a more rewarding and innovative approach both to your professional practice and to your academic studies.

It is important, however, to remember that critical thinking skills need to be developed over time, and do not always come easily. We hope that this book has helped you as you set out on your journey as a critical thinker, in order to enhance your own and others' practice in health and social care in the future.

In summary

In this chapter we have explored why critical thinking is important for developing a broader perspective in your personal, professional and academic life, noting that there is a need for creative and flexible professionals who are able to think critically and respond effectively to rapid change. We have discussed the many changes influencing health and social care in the twenty-first century, and explored how health and social care professionals can respond to these as critical thinkers. We have described the qualities and skills that are needed to think critically from a broader perspective in relation to health and social care. We have also discussed how you can broaden your horizons through networking with professionals and academics in different disciplines, professions and specialist fields.

Key points

1 Thinking critically and taking a broad perspective when analysing theory or practice in relation to health and social care issues can lead to positive developments to your own and others' practice, at local, national and much broader levels, as well as to the development of your academic skills.
2 Health and social care professionals need to be critical thinkers to be able to respond effectively to the rapid changes occurring in the twenty-first century. A broad perspective is required, taking into account the various factors impacting on health and social care at local, regional, national and global levels.
3 There are key qualities and skills which will enable you to take a broader perspective in relation to your practice and your studies – in particular flexibility, creativity and responsiveness to change.

Appendix: useful websites

All websites were accessible at time of printing.

Agree Collaboration. An international collaboration of researchers and policy-makers who seek to improve the quality and effectiveness of clinical practice guidelines by establishing a shared framework for their development, reporting and assessment. www.agreecollaboration.org

Bad Science. Author Ben Goldacre discusses many of the myths about health and social care especially those reported in the media. www.insightassessment. com/pdf_files/What&Why2010.pdf

Bandolier. A useful and easy to read independent journal on evidence-based practice. www.medicine.ox.ac.uk/bandolier

Best Health. An evidence-based patient website, based on the *British Medical Journal*'s Clinical Evidence. It explains chronic conditions and rates the effectiveness of treatments. Subscription is needed for access to some information. http://besthealth.bmj.com/btuk/home.jsp

Center for Health Evidence. A very good set of guides to using the literature were published in the *Journal of the American Medical Association (JAMA)* a few years ago and are now available on the web with clinical scenarios and worked examples of question answering. www.cche.net/principles/content_all.asp

Centre for Evidence Based Medicine (CEBM). The aim is to develop, teach and promote evidence-based health care and provide support and resources to doctors and health care professionals to help maintain the highest standards of medicine. www.cebm.net

Clinical Evidence. One of the world's most authoritative medical resources for informing treatment decisions and improving patient care. http://clinicalevidence.bmj.com/ceweb/index.jsp

Cochrane Collaboration. For systematic reviews, clinical trials and other sources. www.cochrane.org

Critical Appraisal Skills Programme (CASP). Aims to enable individuals to develop the skills to find and make sense of research evidence, helping them to put knowledge into practice. www.sph.nhs.uk/what-we-do/public-health-workforce/resources/critical-appraisals-skills-programme

Critical Thinking Community. An educational, non-profit organization that aims to cultivate fair-minded critical thinking. There are a variety of resources and web links. www.criticalthinking.org/index.cfm

Critical Thinking on the Web. A directory of quality online resources. http://austhink.com/critical/pages/definitions.html

Department of Health. Access to national guidance, benchmarking standards and policy relating to health and social care. www.dh.gov.uk/en/index.htm www.dh.gov.uk/en/SocialCare/index.htm

Evidence-based Answers to Clinical Questions for Busy Clinicians. A workbook published in 2009 by The Centre for Clinical Effectiveness, Southern Health, Melbourne, Australia. www.southernhealth.org.au/icms_docs/2145_EBP_workbook.pdf

Evidence in Health & Social Care. NHS evidence allows everyone working in health and social care to access a wide range of health information to help them deliver quality patient care. www.evidence.nhs.uk/default.aspx

Gavel. An evidence-based medicine publication written specifically for primary care, based on a comprehensive search of the world's literature. Each issue summarizes the clinically important research findings that influence therapeutic choice. http://www.evidence-based-medicine.co.uk/default.html

General Social Care Council (GSCC). http://www.gscc.org.uk

Health Information Research Unit (HIRU). Based at the Clinical Epidemiology and Biostatistics Department at McMaster University, Canada, the Unit conducts research in the field of health information science. http://hiru.mcmaster.ca/hiru

Health Professions Council. www.hpc-uk.org

Internet for Health and Social Care. Designed to help university students develop their internet research skills. www.vtstutorials.ac.uk/tutorial/health-andsocialcare/?sid=2361054&itemid=1202

Intute. Offers a selection of education and research sources by subject area. There is a particular site relating to health and social care. www.intute.ac.uk/healthandlifesciences/nmaplost.html

Joanna Briggs Institute. An international not-for-profit research and development organization specializing in evidence-based resources for health care professionals in nursing, midwifery, medicine and allied health. http://www.joannabriggs.edu.au

Map of Medicine. A clinical information framework designed to make specialized and evidence-based practice readily accessible to non-specialists by tracing the patient journey from the first presentation through to final outcome. http://www.mapofmedicine.com

National Guideline Clearinghouse. A public resource for evidence-based clinical practice guidelines. www.guideline.gov

National Institute for Health and Clinical Excellence (NICE). An independent organization responsible for providing national guidance on promoting good health and preventing and treating ill health. www.nice.org.uk

NHS Centre for Reviews and Dissemination. Based at York University, this includes the Database of Reviews of Effectiveness (DARE), the NHS Economic Evaluation Database (NHS EED) and the Health Technology Assessment Database. www.york.ac.uk/inst/crd

Nursing and Midwifery Council (NMC). www.nmc-uk.org

Pinakes. A useful subject launch pad which offers an approach for identifying sources relating to specific topic areas. www.hw.ac.uk/libwww/irn/pinakes/pinakes.html

Social Care Online. The UK's most complete range of information and research on all aspects of social care. www.scie-socialcareonline.org.uk

What is . . .? A series which explains the terminology and concepts used in evidence-based medicine. www.whatisseries.co.uk/whatis

Glossary

Abstract: A short summary of what a paper is about which is usually printed at the beginning of the paper.

Accountable: To be answerable for your acts and your omissions.

Analysis: Breaking down a concept or an experience into parts.

Anecdotal evidence: Where personal opinion or information not based on proven facts is used as evidence.

Best available evidence: This is evidence that is found through a professional database search. It will depend on the question you are asking.

Case control study: A study in which people with a specific condition (cases) are compared to people without this condition (controls) to compare the frequency of the occurrence of the exposure that might have caused the condition.

Cohort study: A study in which two or more groups or cohorts are followed up to examine whether exposures measured at the beginning lead to outcomes, such as disease.

Confidence interval: Confidence intervals are usually (but arbitrarily) 95 per cent confidence intervals. A reasonable, though strictly incorrect interpretation, is that the 95 per cent confidence interval gives the range in which the population effect lies.

Critical analysis: Where you break down or explore in depth all the information available relating to an issue or question. This may involve exploring what is happening and the reasons why. You may need to consider and access alternative perspectives including theory.

Critical appraisal: Where you consider the strengths and limitations of each piece of evidence you use.

Critical appraisal tool: A checklist or series of prompt questions used to assess the quality of evidence.

Critical thinking: Where you adopt a questioning approach and thoughtful attitude to what you read, see or hear, rather than accepting things at face value. It relates to both academic work and professional practice.

Database: Subject-specific databases hold the references for, and often the abstracts or full text for journal articles and many other texts, for which you can search using key words.

Description: Where information is given (verbally or in writing) in a factual manner.

Descriptive statistics: Statistics such as means, medians and standard deviations that describe aspects of the data, such as central tendency (mean or median) or its dispersion (standard deviation).

Discussion paper: A paper presenting an argument or discussion.

Empirical research: Research which is based on observation or experiment. The opposite is theoretical research.

Ethnography: A qualitative research approach which involves the study of the culture or way of life of participants.

Evaluation: Judging and forming opinion, based on a sound argument – this involves the appraisal of information or evidence.

Evidence-based practice: Practice that is supported by clear reasoning, taking into account the patient's or client's preferences and using your own judgement.

Exclusion criteria: Criteria that are set in order to focus the searching strategy for a literature review (e.g. not children, not acute care episodes, before 2005).

Explanation: When using an explanatory style of writing or presenting, you provide justification or reasons for your actions, views and arguments.

Generalizability: Where the findings from a research study can be applied in other contexts.

Grounded theory: Qualitative research approach that involves the generation of theory.

Hierarchy of evidence: Strong evidence is at the top of the hierarchy and weaker evidence is at the bottom. Classifications as to what counts as strong evidence vary according to what you are trying to find out

Inclusion and exclusion criteria: Criteria that are set in order to focus the searching strategy for a literature review (e.g. research from the past five years, published in English).

Inferential statistics: Statistics that are used to infer findings from the sample population to the wider population, usually meaning statistical tests.

Narrative review: A literature review that is not undertaken according to a predefined and systematic approach.

P values: The p (probability) value is the probability of observing results more extreme than those observed if the null hypothesis was true.

Phenomenology: Qualitative research approach in which the participants 'lived experience' is explored.

Practice assessor/mentor: Those who support learners in practice. A variety of terms are used throughout the professions such as clinical educator, supervisor, practice educator/teacher, clinical tutor or instructor.

Qualitative research: Generally uses interviews to explore the *experience or meaning* of an issue in depth. The results are presented as *words*.

Quantitative research: Generally explores if something is *effective or not*, or is used to measure the *amount of something*. Results are generally presented using *numbers* or *statistics*.

Questionnaires/surveys: Studies in which a sample is taken at *any one point in time* from *a defined group of people* and observed/assessed.

Randomization: The process of allocating individuals randomly to groups (or control groups) in a trial.

Randomized controlled trial (RCT): A trial which has randomly assigned groups in order to determine the effectiveness of an intervention(s) which is given to one or two of the groups.

Rationale: Where you give clear reasons for your practice decisions or actions.

Readily available information: Information that you encounter on an everyday basis and do not need to look too hard to find.

Reflection: Reflection is about reviewing an experience in order to learn from it.

Research methodology: The process undertaken in order to address the research question.

Research question: A question set by researchers at the outset of a study, to be addressed in the study.

Snowballing: A method of finding more literature by looking at the reference lists of papers you have found through a database search.

Students/learners: Anyone, pre- or post-qualifying, who may be undertaking study either formally or informally.

Systematic review: A very detailed literature review that seeks to summarize all available evidence on a topic with clear explanations of the approach taken (methodology). It is the most detailed type of review.

Transferability: In qualitative studies the findings may be used and interpreted by others, although the aim in qualitative research is not to generalize.

References

Action on Smoking and Health (2010) *Smoking Rates: Adults*, www.ashscotland.org.uk/ash/4320, accessed 18 October 2010.

Alcock, P. (2008) *Social Policy in Britain*, 3rd edn. Basingstoke: Palgrave Macmillan

Appleton, J. (2008) Using reflection in a palliative care educational programme, in C. Bulman and S. Schutz (eds) *Reflective Practice in Nursing*, 4th edn. Oxford: Blackwell.

Atkins, S. and Murphy, K. (1993) Reflection: a review of the literature, *Journal of Advanced Nursing*, 29(1): 201–7.

Atkins, S. and Schutz, S. (2008) Developing the skills for reflective practice, in C. Bulman and S. Schutz (eds) *Reflective Practice in Nursing*, 4th edn. Oxford: Blackwell.

Aveyard, H. (2010) *Doing a Literature Review in Health and Social Care*. Maidenhead: Open University Press.

Aveyard, H. and Sharp, P. (2009) *A Beginner's Guide to Evidence Based Practice*. Maidenhead: Open University Press.

Bandura, A. (1965) Influence of models' reinforcement contingencies on the acquisition of imitative responses, *Journal of Personality and Social Psychology*, 1(6): 589–95.

Banning, M. (2008) A review of clinical decision making: models and current research, *Journal of Clinical Nursing*, 17(2): 187–95.

Barnett, R. (2000) *Realizing the University in an Age of Supercomplexity*. Buckingham: SRHE/Open University Press.

Barnett, R. (2004) Learning for an unknown future, *Higher Education Research and Development*, 23(3): 247–56.

Baxter, S. *et al.* (2010) *Systematic Review of How to Stop Smoking in Pregnancy and Following Childbirth*. Sheffield: University of Sheffield School of Health and Related Research.

Bidmead, C. and Cowley, S. (2005) A concept analysis of partnership with clients, *Community Practitioner*, 76(6): 203–8.

Biley, F.C. and Wright, S.G. (1997) Towards a defense of nursing ritual and routine, *Journal of Clinical Nursing*, 6(2): 115–19.

Blakemore, K. and Griggs, E. (2007) *Social Policy: An Introduction*, 3rd edn. Maidenhead: Open University Press.

Bluff, R. and Holloway, I. (2008) The efficacy of midwifery role models, *Midwifery*, 24: 301–9.

Booth, S. (2010) Pregnant and can't give up smoking . . . despite son's pleas and risks to unborn baby, *Daily Record*, 29 June, www.dailyrecord.co.uk/news/real-life/2010/06/29/i-m-pregnant-at-age-40-but-can-t-give-up-cigarettes-86908-22368808, accessed 26 April 2011.

Bourn, D., McKenzie, A. and Shiel, C. (2006) *The Global University: The Role of the Curriculum*. London: Development Education Association.

Bradshaw, T., Butterworth A. and Mairs, H. (2007) Does structured clinical supervision during psychological education enhance outcome for mental health nurses and the service users they work with? *Journal of Psychiatric and Mental Health Nursing*, 14: 4–12.

Bridges, D. (2000) Back to the future: the higher education curriculum in the twenty-first century, *Cambridge Journal of Education*, 30(1): 37–55.

Brookfield, S. (1987) *Developing Critical Thinkers: Challenging Adults to Explore Alternative Ways of Thinking and Acting*. San Francisco: Jossey-Bass.

Brotherton, G. and Parker, S. (2008) *Your Foundation in Health and Social Care*. London: Sage.

Brown, T. *et al.* (2010) Practice education learning environments: the mismatch between perceived and preferred expectations of undergraduate health science students, *Nurse Education Today*, doi:10.1016/j.nedt.2010.11.013.

Bulman, C. and Schutz, S. (2008) *Reflective Practice in Nursing*, 4th edn. Oxford: Blackwell.

Castledine, G. (2010) Critical thinking is crucial, *British Journal of Nursing*, 19(4): 271.

Commission on Social Determinants of Health (2008) *Closing the Gap in a Generation: Health equity through action on the social determinants of Health: Final report of the Commission on Social determinants*. Geneva: World Health Organization.

Cottrell, S. (2005) *Critical Thinking Skills: Developing Effective Argument and Analysis*. Basingstoke: Palgrave Macmillan.

Cottrell, S. (2008) *The Study Skills Handbook*, 3rd edn. London: Palgrave Macmillan.

Cruess, S.R., Cruess, R.L. and Steinert, Y. (2008) Role modelling – making the most of a powerful teaching tool, *British Medical Journal*, 336: 718–21.

Dahlgren, G. and Whitehead, M. (1993) *Policies and Strategies to Promote Health and Social Equity in Europe*. Stockholm: Institute of Futures Studies.

Dahlgren, G. and Whitehead, M. (2007) *European Strategies for Tackling Social Determinants of Inequities in Health: Levelling up Part 2: Studies in Social and Economic Determinants of Population Health*, 3. Copenhagen: European Regional Office of the World Health Organization.

Dawes, M. *et al.* (2005) *Evidence Based Practice: A Primer for Health Care Professionals*. Edinburgh: Churchill Livingstone.

Deer, B, (2011) Secrets of the MMR scare: *The Lancet*'s two days to bury bad news, *British Medical Journal*, 342: c7001.

Department of Health (2009) *Religion or Belief – A Practical Guide for the NHS*. London: Department of Health.

Department of Health (2010) *Healthy Lives, Healthy People: Our Strategy for Public Health in England*. London: Department of Health.

DiCenso, A., Cliliska, D. and Guyatt, G. (eds) (2004) *Evidence Based Nursing: A Guide to Clinical Practice*. St Louis, MO: Elsevier.

Dimond, B. (2008) *Legal Aspects of Nursing*. Harlow: Longman.

Downie, R. and Macnaughton, J. (2009) In defence of professional judgement, *Advances in Psychiatric Treatment*, 15: 322–7.

Drennan, D. (1992) *Transforming Company Culture*. Maidenhead: McGraw-Hill.

Driscoll, J. (2007) *Practising Clinical Supervision: A Reflective Approach for Healthcare Professionals*. Edinburgh: Bailliere Tindall/Elsevier.

Dunphy, L. *et al.* (2010) Reflections and learning from using action learning sets in a healthcare education setting, *Action Learning, Research and Practice*, 7: 303–14.

Facione, P.A. (1990) *Critical Thinking: A Statement of Expert Consensus for Purposes of Educational Assessment and Instruction. Executive Summary 'The Delphi Report'*. Millbrae, CA: The California Academic Press.

Facione, P.A. (2011a) Critical thinking: what it is and why it counts, *Insight Assessment*, 1–28, www.insightassessment.com/pdf_files/What&Why2010.pdf, accessed 20 April 2011.

Facione, P.A. (2011b) *Think Critically*. Englewood Cliffs, NJ: Pearson Education.

Facione, P.A., Facione, N.C. and Giancarlo, C.A.F. (1997) *Professional Judgment and the Dispostition Toward Critical Thinking*. Millbrae, CA: California Academic Press.

Flanagan, J.C. (1954) The critical incident technique, *Psychological Bulletin*, 51(4): 327–59.

Fraser, A.G. and Dunstan, F.D. (2010) On the impossibility of being expert, *British Medical Journal*, 341: c7126.

Gabbay, J. and Le May, A. (2004) Evidence based guidelines or collectively constructed 'mindlines?' Ethnographic study of knowledge management in primary care, *British Medical Journal*, 329: 1013.

Gallacher, J. and Osborne, M. (2005) *A Contested Landscape: International Perspectives on Diversity in Mass Higher Education*. Leicester: National Institute for Adult and Continuing Education (NIACE).

Geleijnse, J.M., Brouwer, I.A. and Feskens, E.J.M. (2006) Risks and benefits of omega 3 fats: health benefits of omega 3 fats are in doubt, *British Medical Journal*, 332: 915.

General Social Care Council (GSCC) (2010) *Codes of Practice for Employers of Social Care Workers*. London: GSCC.

Gibbs, G. (1988) *Learning by Doing: A Guide to Teaching and Learning Methods*. Oxford: Further Education Unit, Oxford Polytechnic.

Gill, C.J. *et al.* (2011) Effect of training traditional birth attendants on neonatal mortality, *British Medical Journal*, 432: 373.

Goldacre, B. (2009) *Bad Science*. London: Harper Perennial.

Green Lister, P. and Crisp, B.R. (2007) Critical incident analysis: a practice learning tool for students and practitioners, *Practice: Social Work in Action*, 19(1): 47–60.

Griffiths, R. and Tengnah, C. (2008) *Law and Professional Nursing*. Poole: Learning Matters.

Gross Forneris, S. and Peden-McAlpine, C. (2009) Creating context for critical thinking in practice, the role of the preceptor, *Journal of Advanced Nursing*, 65(8): 1715–24.

Halvorsen, T. (2008) How to quit smoking during pregnancy: tips to stop smoking, www.howtodothings.com/family-and-relationships/a2621-how-to-quit-smoking-during-pregnancy.html, accessed 26 April 2011.

Harrison, G. and Melville, R. (2010) *Rethinking Social Work in a Global World* Basingstoke: Palgrave Macmillan.

Health Professions Council (HPC) (2008) *Standards for Conduct Performance and Ethics*. London: HPC.

Hek, G., Judd, M. and Moule, P. (2003) *Making Sense of Research: An Introduction for Health & Social Care Professionals*, 2nd edn. London: Sage.

Held, D., McGrew, A., Goldblatt, D. and Perraton, J. (1999) What is globalization? www.polity.co.uk/global/whatisglobalization.asp, accessed 20 April 2011.

Helms, M.M. and Nixon, J. (2010) Exploring SWOT analysis – where are we now? A review of academic research from the last decade, *Journal of Strategy and Management*, 3(3): 215–51.

Higgs, J. and Hunt, A. (1999) Rethinking the beginning practitioner: introducing the 'interactional professional', in J. Higgs and H. Edwards (eds) *Educating Beginning Practitioners: Challenges for Professional Education*. Melbourne: Butterworth Heinemann.

Higher Education Academy/Health Sciences and Practice (2005) *Health Sciences and Practice: Nursing Student Employability Profile*. London: Higher Education Academy/ Health Sciences and Practice.

Holland, K. (2010) Culture, race and ethnicity: exploring the concepts in K. Holland and C. Hogg (2010) *Cultural Awareness in Nursing and Health Care: An Introductory Text*, 2nd edn. London: Hodder Arnold.

Hopper L. *et al.* (2006) Risks and benefits of omega 3 fats for mortality, cardiovascular disease, and cancer: systematic review, *British Medical Journal*, 332: 752–60.

Huckabay, L.M. (2009) Clinical reasoned judgment and the nursing process, *Nursing Forum*, 44(2): 72–8.

Iles, V. and Sutherland, K. (2004) *Organisational Change: A Review for Healthcare Managers, Professionals and Researchers.* London: National Coordinating Centre for Service Delivery and Organisation.

Information Centre (2006) *Statistics on Smoking: England, 2006*, http://www.ic.nhs.uk/webfiles/publications/smokingeng2006/Smoking%20bulletin%202006%20-%20Finalv3.pdf, accessed 26 April 2011.

Jasper, M. (2007) *Reflection, Decision Making and Professional Development.* Oxford: Blackwell.

Jasper, M. (2008) Using reflective journals and diaries to enhance practice and learning, in C. Bulman and S. Schutz (eds) *Reflective Practice in Nursing*, 4th edn. Oxford: Blackwell.

Johns, C. and Freshwater, D. (2005) *Transforming Nursing Through Reflective Practice*, 2nd edn. Oxford: Blackwell.

Kadushin, A. and Harkness, D. (2002) *Supervision in Social Work*, 4th edn. New York: Columbia University Press.

Kamhi, A.G. (2011) Balancing uncertainty and uncertainty in clinical practice, *Language, Speech and Hearing in Schools*, 15: 226–34.

Keene, E.A., Hutton, N., Hall, B. and Ruston, C. (2010) Bereavement debriefing sessions: an intervention to support health care professionals in managing their grief after the death of a patient, *Pediatric Nursing*, 36(4): 185–9.

Kida, T. (2006) *Don't Believe Everything You Think: The Six Basic Mistakes We Make in Thinking.* Amherst, NY: Prometheus.

Lumley, J. *et al.* (2009) Interventions for promoting smoking cessation during pregnancy, *Cochrane Database of Systematic Reviews*, 3, www2.cochrane.org/reviews/en/ab001055.html, accessed 26 April 2011.

Mann, K., Gordon, J. and MacLeod, A. (2009) Reflection and reflective practice in health professions: a systematic review, *Advances in Health Science Education*, 14: 595–621.

McCarthy, J. and Rose P. (2010) *Values-based Health & Social Care: Beyond Evidence-based Practice.* London: Sage.

McGill, I. and Beaty, L. (2001) *Action Learning: A Guide for Professional, Management and Educational Development.* Oxford: Routledge Farmer.

McMahon, R. and Pearson, A. (1998) *Nursing as Therapy*, 2nd edn. London: Stanley Thornes.

Melhuish, E., Belsky, J. and Leyland, A .(2010) *The Impact of Sure Start Local Programmes on Five Year Olds and Their Families.* London: Birkbeck University of London/Department of Education, www.ness.bbk.ac.uk/impact/documents/RR067.pdf.

Moon, J. (1999) *Reflection in Learning and Professional Development.* London: Kogan Page.

Moyer, V.A. and Elliott, E.J. (2004) *Evidenced Based Pediatrics and Child Health*, 2nd edn. London: British Medical Journal Books.

Myrick, F. and Yonge, O. (2002) Preceptor behaviors integral to the promotion of student critical thinking, *Journal for Nurses in Staff Development*, 18(3): 127–33.

National Institute for Health and Clinical Excellence (NICE) (2010) *Quitting Smoking in Pregnancy and Following Childbirth: Quick Reference Guide.* London: NICE.

National Statistics (2006) *Statistics on NHS Stop Smoking Services in England, 2006*, www.ic.nhs.uk/webfiles/publications/smokingeng2006/StatisticsOnSmoking300806_PDF.pdf, accessed 26 April 2011.

Newton, J.M., Jolly, B.C., Ockerby, C.M. and Cross, W.M. (2010) Clinical learning environment inventory: factor analysis, *Journal of Advanced Nursing*, 66(6): 1371–81.

Nursing and Midwifery Council (NMC) (2008) *The Code: Standards for Conduct, Performance and Ethics for Nurses and Midwives*. London: NMC.

Nursing and Midwifery Council (NMC) (2010) *Raising and Escalating Concerns: Guidance for Nurses and Midwives*. London: NMC.

O'Connell, N. (2009) Smoking cessation management must become more individualised, *Nurse Prescribing*, 7(11): 486–8.

Olsen, D. (2000) Editorial comment, *Nursing Ethics*, 7(6): 470–1.

Paul, R. and Elder, L. (2005) *Critical Thinking: Tools for Taking Charge of Your Professional and Personal Life*. Upper Saddle River, NJ: Prentice Hall.

Pearson, M. and Smith, D. (1986) Debriefing in experience-based learning, *Simulation/Games for Learning*, 16(4): 155–72.

Petrovic, M., Roberts, R. and Ramsay, M. (2001) Second dose of measles, mumps, and rubella vaccine: questionnaire survey of health professionals, *British Medical Journal*, 322: 82–5.

Phillips, R.S. and Glasziou, P. (2004) What makes evidence based journal clubs succeed? *Evidence Based Medicine*, 9: 36–7.

Price, B. and Harrington, A. (2010) *Critical Thinking and Writing for Nursing Students* Exeter: Learning Matters Ltd.

Reid, B. (1993) 'But we're doing it already': exploring a response to the concept of reflective practice in order to improve its facilitation, *Nurse Education Today*, 13: 305–9.

Seedhouse, D. (2009) *Ethics: The Heart of Healthcare*, 3rd edn. Chichester: Wiley.

Seifert, P.C. (2010) Thinking critically, *AORN Journal*, 91(2): 197–9.

Shipton, T. *et al.* (2009) Reliability of self reported smoking status by pregnant women for estimating smoking prevalence: a retrospective, cross sectional study, *British Medical Journal*, 339:b4347 doi:10.1136/bmj.b4347.

Simpson, E. and Courtney, M. (2002) Critical thinking in nursing education: literature review, *International Journal of Nursing Practice*, 8(2): 89–98.

Smith, G. and Pell, J. (2003) Parachute use to prevent death and major trauma: a systematic review, *British Medical Journal*, 327: 1439.

Smith, R. (2010) Strategies for coping with information overload, *British Medical Journal*, 341: c7126.

Social Care Institute for Excellence (SCIE) (2004) *Learning Organisations: A Self-assessment Resource Pack*, www.scie.org.uk/publications/learningorgs/index.asp, accessed 31 May 2011.

Starr, F. (2001) *Unwrapped: My Autobiography*. London: Virgin.

Stephenson, S. (1994) Reflection – a student's perspective, in A. Palmer, S. Burns and C. Bulman (eds) *Reflective Practice in Nursing: The Growth of the Professional Practitioner*. Oxford: Blackwell Science.

Sterling, S. (2001) *Sustainable Education: Re-visioning Learning and Change*. Totnes: Green Books.

Stillwell, S.B., Finehout-Overholt, E., Mazurek, B. and Williamson, K. (2010) Evidence-based Practice, Step by Step; Asking the Clinical Question: A Key Step in Evidence-Based Practice *American Journal of Nursing*. 110 (3): 58–61.

Sustainable Development Commission (2008) *Health, Place and Nature: How Outdoor Environments Influence Health and Wellbeing – A Knowledge Base*. London: Sustainable Development Commission.

Swann, B. (2002) An effective placement: creating an learning environment, in I. Welsh and C. Swann (eds) *Partners in Learning: A Guide to Support and Assessment in Nursing*. Oxford: Radcliffe Medical Press.

Taylor, B.J. (2006) *Reflective Practice: A Guide for Nurses and Midwives*, 2nd edn. Maidenhead: Open University Press.

Thompson, C. (2003) Clinical experience as evidence in evidence-based practice, *Journal of Advanced Nursing*, 43(3): 230–7.

Turner, P. and Whitfield, T.W.A. (2006) Physiotherapist's use of evidence based practice – a cross-national study, *Physiotherapy Research International*, 2(1): 17–29.

United Nations (1987) *Report of the World Commission on Environment and Development General Assembly Resolution 42/187, 11 December 1987*. Oxford: Oxford University.

United Nations (2009) *World Population Ageing 2009*, www.un.org/esa/population/publications/WPA2009/WPA2009-report.pdf, accessed 17 April 2011.

United Nations Environment Programme/WHO (2008) *Libreville Declaration on Health and Environment in Africa*. Libreville: World Health Organization Regional Office for Africa.

University of Leicester (2010) *What is Critical Writing?* www2.le.ac.uk/offices/ssds/sd/ld/resources/writing/writing-resources/critical-writing.

Wade, C. and Tarvis, C. (2008) *Psychology*, 9th edn. Upper Saddle River, NJ: Prentice Hall.

Wakefield, A.J., Murch, S.H., Anthony, A. and Linnell, J. (1998) Ileal-lymphoid-nodular hyperplasia, non-specific colitis and pervasive developmental disorder in children, *The Lancet*, 351.637–41 (paper now withdrawn).

Wellington, J. *et al.* (2005) *Succeeding with your Doctorate*. London: Sage.

Welsh, I. and Swann, C. (eds) (2002) *Partners in Learning: A Guide to Support and Assessment in Nursing*. Oxford: Radcliffe Medical Press.

Williams, C. and Johnson, R.D. (2010) *Race and Ethnicity in a Welfare Society*. Maidenhead: Open University Press.

Woolliams, M. (2007) The incorporation of global perspectives into the higher professional education of healthcare professionals: an analysis of the intentions of teachers in relation to student learning, unpublished MSc dissertation, Oxford Brookes University School of Health and Social Care.

Woolliams, M., Williams, K., Butcher, D. and Pye, D. (2009) *Be More Critical! A Practical Guide for Health and Social Care Students*. Oxford: Oxford Brookes University.

World Health Organization (WHO) (2009) *Phase V (2009–2013) of the WHO European Healthy Cities Network: Goals and Requirements*. Copenhagen: World Health Organization.

World Health Organization (WHO) (2011) *10 Facts on Preventing Disease from Healthy Environments*, www.who.int/features/factfiles/environmental_health/environmental_health_facts/en/index5.htmlaccessed 17 April 2011.

Zisberg, A., Young, H.M., Schepp, K. and Zysberg, L. (2007) A concept analysis of routine: relevance to nursing, *Journal of Advanced Nursing*, 57(4): 442–53.

Index

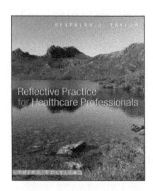

REFLECTIVE PRACTICE FOR HEALTHCARE PROFESSIONALS
Third Edition

Beverley J. Taylor

9780335238354 (Paperback)
2010

eBook also available

This popular book provides practical guidance for healthcare professionals wishing to reflect on their work and improve the way they undertake clinical procedures, interact with other people at work and deal with power issues. The new edition has been broadened in focus from nurses and midwives exclusively, to include all healthcare professionals.

Key features:

- Identifies the fundamentals of reflective practice and how and why it is embraced in healthcare professions
- Includes strategies for effective reflection
- Provides a step-by-step guide to applying the Taylor REFLECT model

www.openup.co.uk

OPEN UNIVERSITY PRESS
McGraw - Hill Education

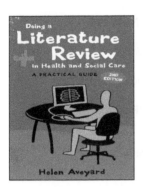

**DOING A LITERATURE REVIEW
IN HEALTH AND SOCIAL CARE
A Practical Guide
Second Edition**

Helen Aveyard

9780335238859 (Paperback)
2010

eBook also available

This bestselling book is a step-by-step guide to doing a literature review in health and social care. It is vital reading for all those undertaking their undergraduate or postgraduate dissertation or any research module which involves a literature review.

The new edition has been fully updated and provides a practical guide to the different types of literature that you may be encountered when undertaking a literature review.

Key features:

- Includes examples of commonly occurring real life scenarios encountered by students
- Provides advice on how to follow a clearly defined search strategy
- Details a wide range of critical appraisal tools that can be utilised

www.openup.co.uk

OPEN UNIVERSITY PRESS
McGraw - Hill Education

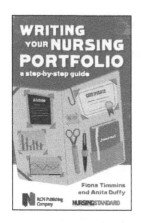

WRITING YOUR NURSING PORTFOLIO
A Step-by-step Guide

Fiona Timmins and Anita Duffy

9780335242849 (Paperback)
April 2011

eBook also available

This book is perfect for nurses who need to do a portfolio and don't know where to start. It explains simply what a portfolio can and cannot include, gives examples of good and bad pieces and demystifies the portfolio for the busy nurse. This is an essential purchase for qualified nurses doing PREP, and those studying who need a portfolio for assessment.

Key features:

- Provides suggested activities and tasks that can be completed and put into a portfolio
- Written as a 'step by step' guide
- Answers all the common questions nurses have about writing their portfolio

www.openup.co.uk

OPEN UNIVERSITY PRESS
McGraw - Hill Education